Mental disorder and legal control

PHILIP BEAN

Senior Lecturer, Department of Social Administration and Social Work, University of Nottingham

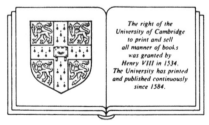

The right of the University of Cambridge to print and sell all manner of books was granted by Henry VIII in 1534. The University has printed and published continuously since 1584.

CAMBRIDGE UNIVERSITY PRESS

Cambridge

New York   New Rochelle

Melbourne   Sydney

CAMBRIDGE UNIVERSITY PRESS
Cambridge, New York, Melbourne, Madrid, Cape Town, Singapore, São Paulo, Delhi

Cambridge University Press
The Edinburgh Building, Cambridge CB2 8RU, UK

Published in the United States of America by Cambridge University Press, New York

www.cambridge.org
Information on this title: www.cambridge.org/9780521102865

First published 1986
Reprinted 1988
This digitally printed version 2009

A catalogue record for this publication is available from the British Library

Library of Congress Cataloguing in Publication data

Bean, Philip.
Mental disorder and legal control.
Includes index.
1. Mental health laws–Great Britain. 2. Insane–
Commitment and detention–Great Britain. I. Title.
[DNLM: 1. Great Britain. Mental Health Act 1983.
2. Mental Disorders–rehabilitation–Great Britain–
legislation. 3. Mental Health Services–Great
Britain–legislation. 4. Patient Advocacy–Great
Britain–legislation. WM 33 FA1 B367m]
KD3412.B42   1986   344.41′044   86-6115
                       344.10444

ISBN 978-0-521-30209-8 hardback
ISBN 978-0-521-10286-5 paperback

Mental disorder and legal control

of the

te

For our son Lee

CONTENTS

PREFACE

These essays are offered from the perspective of a social scientist. They are concerned with the 1983 Mental Health Act as it applies to England and Wales, with its likely effects and its application. The areas covered, although not exhaustive include the major aspects of the legislation; that is they include the compulsory admission procedure for non-offender patients, police powers, guardianship, consent to treatment, offender patients, guardianship and rights of the patient generally. Whilst not intending to be a comparative study as such, it is hoped the essays will highlight some of the issues which are universal and identify questions which are common throughout.

The essays are concerned with specific topics derived from the legislation and complete in themselves. That is, a chapter can be independent of the other chapters with the exception of Chapter 1 which sets the parameters and defines the terms. Thematically the book is concerned with one piece of legislation where in each chapter certain basic questions are asked; for example: what does the legislation say on this topic? What are the implications sociologically and otherwise for the patient, for psychiatry and for society generally? Whilst there are many admirable texts on the legal aspects of this piece of legislation, (see Hoggett, B., 1984 *Mental Health Law*, published by Sweet & Maxwell) and many legal guides, the attempt here is to widen the subject of debate and be less concerned with specific legal issues or with those affecting the day to day management of the patient.

The book is divided into three parts. After the introductory chapter, Section I is entitled 'The admission of patients to mental hospitals' and includes three chapters; one on the medical practitioners, the other on the social workers and the third on the police. Section II, entitled 'Control of patients in the hospital and community' deals with, amongst other things, the mentally abnormal offender and guardianship. Section III deals with patients' rights and includes consent to treatment, legal redress in the courts, and rights related to the Mental Health Act generally. There is also a short concluding chapter.

It would have been possible, I suppose, for these essays to have been written by separate authors. To have done so would have doubtless increased their quality. On the other hand an element of continuity would have been lost, for books of this nature written by different authors coming from different academic traditions make it sometimes difficult for the reader to pick up the threads and for authors to show the extent of their interests. Hopefully whatever is lost in quality in this book is made up for in continuity. These essays are written by someone with no axe to grind other than a deeply held belief that all groups, occupational or otherwise, which have exemplary powers should have their activities carefully scrutinised. That, plus an interest in the subject itself, linked to the view that a study of how we deal with certain selected groups (in this case the mentally disordered) provides insights into the nature of our society generally.

It is my great pleasure to thank those who have assisted throughout. That many people have been prepared to give up their time and energies is a source of comfort and amazement. They are too numerous to mention and it would be invidious to single out a few from the many. There is another group however with whom I am more personally associated which can be mentioned. Mrs Ann Hodson typed the manuscript with her usual efficiency, William Bingley, Irene Overstone and Gillian Pascall kindly read the drafts and made valuable comments. My wife Valerie provided more assistance than anyone could reasonably expect as did our children Ian and Lee. That this book is dedicated to one is to fulfill a promise made years ago and that this is now Lee's turn to receive a dedication.

Philip Bean

CHAPTER 1

Mental Health Legislation

Opportunities to make substantive changes in mental health legislation occur infrequently. In England and Wales the 1890 Lunacy Act confirmed and established legalism; that is, admissions to mental hospitals and treatment in those hospitals were to be governed at all times by statute and controlled and supervised by government bodies such as the Board of Control. The emphasis was on the legal rights of the patient (see Bean, 1980). When legalism was found to be unworkable, mainly because of the stigma said to be associated with mental hospital admissions and the manner in which legalism prevented patients entering mental hospitals except by the courts, the 1930 Mental Treatment Act was introduced. That Act allowed some patients to enter hospital voluntarily, that is without certification. Thirty years later legalism was swept away, to be replaced by a medical view of mental disorder, the terms and definition of which were provided by the Royal Commission preceding the 1959 Mental Health Act (HMSO, 1957). That commission saw mental disorder generally and mental illness in particular as being the province of the medical profession. It was, said the commission, the task of the medical profession to diagnose and treat such conditions and inappropriate for the lawyer and the courts to impose and dictate their terms of reference. The commission's view has now been refined. In the manner in which the 1930 Mental Treatment Act softened legalism, so the 1983 Mental Health Act has softened the medical view. If the history of mental health legislation is anything to go by, England and Wales ought not to expect new legislation before the end of the century, although it appears organisations such as MIND are eager to promote changes at a rather faster rate.

To talk of the medical view of mental disorder is to talk generally. The 1959 Mental Health Act (called the 1959 Act from now on) represented the medical view, yet sustained the powers of the courts in some areas of the civil commitment procedure. Indeed, the Royal commission preceding the 1959 Act (The Percy Commission) spent a considerable time justifying the use of legal powers (see Bean, 1985). When we talk of the medical view, or the medical model, we are talking of a view which was dominant rather than exclusive. To use such terms is to claim a form of academic licence or academic convenience. In this context the medical view means support for the statement of intent made by the Percy Commission; that is mental illness is an illness like any other, that mental patients should be admitted to mental hospitals (or their equivalent) on the basis of psychiatric diagnosis rather than on the decision of the courts, that treatment is primarily if not solely a matter of clinical judgment, and the method and means of detention (where required) is also primarily a clinical matter. In contrast, to say that the 1983 Mental Health Act (called the 1983 Act from now on) or indeed other comparable legislation represents legalism is to say that one or more of those features described above is controlled by statute emphasising the legal rights of the patient.

The 1983 Act has had a short but eventful history (details of which are given in a note at the end of this volume).[1] It was influenced by the recommendations of a number of government committees, notably the Report of the Committee on Mentally Abnormal Offenders (HMSO, 1975) (The Butler Report) and the judgment of the European Commission of Human Rights on 5 November 1980 (X v. United Kingdom) together with various research reports and the activities of certain influential pressure groups, notably MIND (National Association for Mental Health). The 1983 Act is a consolidating Act, having been preceded by the 1982 Mental Health (Amendment) Act. It has been followed by numerous Government Regulations, some of which will be cited throughout, and by Codes of Practice from the newly formed Mental Health Act Commission. At the time of writing (1985) most of the regulations have come into operation, as have a few Codes of Practice.

The Act does not seek to produce new principles, rather it seeks to alter those contained in the 1959 Act. The Parliamentary Under-Secretary of State made such a point, and worth quoting in full.

The Mental Health Act 1959 was a landmark in the development of care for the mentally disordered. It established many important principles. Among them are those which require that where care and treatment in hospital are needed they are given upon a voluntary basis wherever that is possible and that in those few cases where compulsion does prove necessary it must be subject to strict controls. I doubt whether anyone would challenge those principles today; this Bill seeks to amend the 1959 Act but it does not challenge those principles. On the contrary it seeks to ensure that they are more perfectly implemented.

> Parliamentary Debates (1.12.1981), p. 933.

What changes have then taken place? According to Lord Elton, the Parliamentary Under-Secretary of State, they are as follows:

> ... that except in particular circumstances people should not be admitted to detention for treatment in hospital if their condition is not treatable; the provision of much more frequent access to mental health review tribunals; the more stringent regulations of the use of treatment without the consent of the patient; the institution of a special health authority, with particular responsibility to oversee the powers to detain and treat patients under the Act; the institution of interim hospital orders, the powers to remand to hospital for assessment; and I think the limitations of the powers of a guardian to apply only to people over 16 years of age ...

> Parliamentary Debates. (1.12.1981), p.935.

That seems to be a fair summary of the Act and of the government's intentions. Where modifications have occurred, they have as a general rule been with a bias to the rights of the patient. This is not entirely true, for some changes have been made which benefit the professionals to the detriment of the patient. Some changes seem entirely neutral; that is, they are aimed at improving an administrative system. There are some changes where it is claimed the patient will benefit yet as far as I can see, do nothing of the sort; they may even make matters worse. (for example, procedures which allow nursing staff to detain informal patients, see Chapter 3). Perhaps a pastiche of effects was to be expected, for legislation is never likely to satisfy everyone.

Mental health legislation in England and Wales is widely based. It includes those (who we can call patients from now on, to make it easier; and, for convenience sake, we can also refer to the patients as male) who would fit into the broad rubric of the mentally disordered. It includes too such matters as the patient's right to vote, the administration of mental health services, and the removal of patients overseas. Generally speaking, the legislation is concerned with two basic questions: first, how should patients and staff (that is, medical and allied workers) be regulated in the manner in which patients make contact with psychiatric services; second, how should patients and staff be regulated in the manner in which psychiatric treatment is provided. These are timeless questions yet are required periodically to be updated and reviewed according to changes in contemporary conditions. In the first the government said it aimed to provide as much opportunity as possible for patients to seek treatment on a voluntary basis. Where voluntary treatment is not forthcoming then, subject to certain conditions (and including offenders and non-offenders alike) compulsory treatment should by provided. In the second, that is in the manner in which the extent and type of treatment provided should be regulated, the Act attempts to balance the demands of the patient's condition with the types of treatment to be imposed.

All societies are faced with these questions and all answer them in their own fashioh. In England and Wales non-offender patients are compulsorily admitted as a result of medical recommendations together with an application from a social worker or a relative. Some countries use the courts, others not. In England and Wales some limits are imposed on the clinical freedom of the medical profession, elsewhere this is different. There does not appear to be a pattern, or perhaps even a logic, in the way societies operate; those insisting that the court should determine admission, on the grounds that liberty can only be taken by the judiciary, appear not to see it as important to restrict clinical freedom. Some countries mix offender and non-offender patients in the same system, others not. Of course things are not as haphazard as this, though they may appear so to the outsider. Each society grapples with the problems in its own way, some dictated by the availability of resources, others affected by geographical factors and so on. The provision of mental health services in remote areas of Canada, for example, places burdens which do not exist in a densely populated urban society in England and Wales. In some Third World countries, primary psychiatric care does not exist, and complex mental health legislation becomes somewhat inappropriate. In England and Wales, which has a long history of mental health legislation, historical precedents have been created and built up, mixed with a tradition where the types of services produce a unique national flavour. To understand why, say, social workers are involved in compulsory admissions in England and Wales we need look to the origin of social work. The same is true of guardianship and so on.

We can go some way towards answering the first question, that is the manner in which patients make contact with the psychiatrist, by asking about the legal classification of patients. That is, who are the patients under the 1983 Act and how does that legislation classify them? The second major question is much wider and will be dealt with throughout many of the chapters that follow, more particularly in Sections II and III.

Types of patients

England and Wales, in common with many other countries, have experienced a steep decline in the numbers of compulsory patients and of beds in mental hospitals. There has been a drop in aggregate and percentage of compulsory admissions for non-offender patients from about 19% in 1960 to about 10.1% in 1979 (DHSS, 1981). The trend is downward except for patients detained under Section 136 of the 1983 Act; that is where a police constable detains someone deemed to be suffering from mental disorder in a public place (see Chapter 4). Some details of inpatients at one hospital are given at the end of this chapter.[2] Alongside this, at the end of 1954, there were 344 beds per 100 000 of the population; this was halved to 171 per 100 000 by 1978. The total number of mental hospital beds was reduced from 160 000 to 80 000 during the same period. This reduction was due in part to the discharge of certain long-stay patients but, to a greater extent, to a decrease in the patients' average length of stay (Roth, 1985).

To speak of formal and informal admissions in this way where one is contrasted with the other is misleading. I deal with this point in greater detail later (in Chapter 3). For the present however two points can be made; first in my view, Thomas Szasz is entirely correct when he says the presence of legal controls makes a mockery of the term voluntary, for legal controls can always be used as a threat to secure a voluntary admission (Szasz, 1970). (The ancient Latin phrase *coactus voluit*, 'at his will although coerced', sums it up nicely.) Second, there are some patients (the mentally impaired child or the demented elderly) who may not be admitted under a formal order but whose detention is equally real. That they may not require a formal order matters little, for being unaware of their surroundings and unable to do anything about it makes the order unnecessary. It does not alter their predicament. That only 3% of the mentally impaired are formally detained may, on the face of it, appear satisfactory but only if one sees detention in formal legal terms. It takes no account of the social reality of these patients.

Moreover to speak of a drop in the number of hospital beds is also misleading for it could imply that the mental hospital was the sole institution for the detention and treatment of the mentally disordered. Yet not everyone in the mental hospital is disordered, and not all the disordered are in a mental hospital. Mentally disordered patients are dispersed throughout other institutions, whether they be prisons, the so-called special hospitals (by that I mean those hospitals which are controlled by the Secretary of State where admission is only by approval of the Secretary of State, see Chapter 6), and even old peoples' homes. To illustrate this point consider the research study conducted by Dr Irene Ovenstone and myself on admissions to old peoples' homes in Nottingham in 1977 (Ovenstone & Bean, 1981).

A total of 272 people were admitted of whom 117 (or 43%) were from the local geriatric hospitals and 155 (or 57%) from the community. All were

Residents admitted to old peoples' homes in Nottingham and their medical, psychiatric and behavioural assesssment[a]

	Patients ($N = 272$)	
	Admitted from hospital	Admitted from the community
Per cent (and number) of total	43(117)	57(155)
Per cent (and number) who had undiscovered medical condition on admission	44(51)	81(126)
Diagnosis of psychiatric condition: per cent (and number)		
Dementia	56(66)	48(74)
Functional mental illnesses	16(19)	14(22)
Mixed conditions	7(8)	12(19)
No psychiatric condition	21(24)	26(40)
Total	100(117)	100(155)
Behavioural assessment for both groups: percent (and number)		
Severely disabled	6(16)	
Moderately disabled	77(210)	
Independent	17(46)	
Total	100(272)	

[a]I am grateful to the *British Journal of Psychiatry* for granting permission to reproduce these data.

given extensive medical and psychiatric examinations together with a thorough behavioural assessment. The results are best illustrated by a table (above).

That 79% of those admitted from hospital and 74% from the community were diagnosed as having a psychiatric condition illustrates the point that many mental patients, or patients suffering from mental conditions are elsewhere than in mental hospital. (That 44% had undiscovered medical conditions, and those of a serious nature, who were admitted from hospitals says much of the quality of care in general hospitals!) Bearing in mind that old peoples' homes were designed to cater for the eldery in a manner like that received by those who wished to pay for their care, it is not suprising then that old peoples' homes have never been equipped or staffed to deal with the mentally disordered. There were 17 homes, each catering for between 45 and 50 residents, in three of the homes there were three qualified nursing staff, in four there were two, and in the remainder none at all. From the data given above it is clear that old peoples' homes have become surrogate psychogeriatric hospitals, and that they lack the necessary facilities to perform their newly acquired role. We may say with some degree of satisfaction that the long-stay patients in mental hospitals are living in less overcrowded conditions than hitherto but this may have been achieved by causing other institutions to take mental patients. A detailed study of these auxiliary institutions is long overdue; the evidence suggests that more mentally disordered are living in less-than-suitable conditions, receiving less-than-adequate care. This point of course is often made by critics of contemporary forms of community care (see Scull, 1983). What is given less attention however is the mode of referral. That a patient should go to an old peoples' home rather than elsewhere seems often to be a matter of chance and the facilities available at the time rather than part of a coordinated public policy.

Legal classifications

The architects of the 1983 Act spent a great deal of parliamentary time debating the nature and types of mental disorder. Sadly their deliberations have hardly led to an improvement, some critics believing that things are worse now than before. No doubt the complexity of the subject matter made it difficult to provide adequate legal definitions but, even so, some definitions verge on the tautological and others are pedantic and obscure. Here I wish to describe the legal terminology rather than to examine it in detail, for the aim is to provide the necessary platform for later discussions.

To summarise: the Act makes two distinctions. First, the generic term 'mental disorder' is used where admission is for assessment (Sections 2 or 4) or the patient is to be removed to a place of safety (Sections 135 or 136). For those sections providing for longer periods of detention, the Act requires that the patient must have one of the four specific forms of mental disorder: that is, mental illness, mental impairment, severe mental impairment or psychopathic disorder. Second, and over and above this, the specific forms of mental disorder can themselves be further classified into major and minor types of disorders: the major ones being mental illness and severe mental impairment which justify admission even if hospital treatment is unlikely to do the patient good, while the minor disorders of psychopathic disorder and mental impairment justify admission only if treatment is likely to make the patient better, or (if not) then to stop him from getting worse.

The definitions are contained in Section 1. Section 1(2) says

In this Act –
'Mental disorder' means mental illness, arrested or incomplete development of mind, psychopathic disorder and any other disorder or disability of mind and 'mentally disordered' shall be construed accordingly:
'Severe mental impairment' means a state of arrested or incomplete development of

mind which includes severe impairment of intelligence and social functioning and is associated with abnormally aggressive or seriously irresponsible conduct on the part of the person concerned and 'severely mentally impaired' shall be construed accordingly;

'mental impairment' means a state of arrested or incomplete development of mind (not amounting to severe mental impairment) which includes significant impairment of intelligence and social functioning and is associated with abnormally aggressive or seriously irresponsible conduct on the part of the person concerned, and 'mentally impaired' shall be construed accordingly;

'psychopathic disorder' means a persistent disorder of disability of mind (whether or not including significant impairment or intelligence) which results in abnormally aggressive or seriously irresponsible conduct on the part of the person concerned;

Section 1(3) adds a caveat.

Nothing in subsection (2) above shall be construed as implying that a person may be dealt with under this Act as suffering from mental disorder, or from any form of mental disorder described in this section by reason only of promiscuity or other immoral conduct, sexual deviancy or dependence on alcohol or drugs.

Mental illness, one of the major forms of mental disorder is not therefore defined in the 1983 Act nor was it under the 1959 Act. The current omission is regrettable. It represents a lost opportunity which would have forced greater attention on the nature of the psychiatric task. As things now stand there remains the suspicion that mental illness defies definition, needlessly providing the sceptics and the anti-psychiatrists with much to cling to.[3] For, in spite of imperfections, the DHSS had earlier produced a definition which could have formed the basis of further discussions and possibly been included in the legislation. The DHSS said mental illness means an illness having one or more of the following classifications:

(i)   more than temporary impairment of intellectual functions shown by a failure of memory, orientation, comprehension or learning capacity;

(ii)   more than a temporary alteration of mood of such degree as to give rise to the patient having a delusional appraisal of his situation, his past or his future or that of others or to the lack of any appraisal;

(iii)   delusional beliefs, persecutory, jealous or grandiose;

(iv)   abnormal perspectives associated with delusional misinterpretations of events;

(v)   thinking so disordered as to prevent the patient making a reasonable appraisal or having reasonable communication with others DHSS (1976).

This definition is not without its flaws yet it remains superior to many others currently available. The Butler Committee, for example, defined mental illness as 'a disorder which has not always existed in the patient but has developed as a condition overlying the sufferer's personality' (HMSO, 1975, para. 1.13). In Canada (Alberta) mental illness includes alcoholism, and in the USA (Indiana) it includes mental retardation, epilepsy, alcoholism and addiction to narcotic and dangerous drugs (Curran & Harding, T. 1978, p 36). It is also superior to the definition found in case law where Lawton (L. J.) said the term mental illness had 'no legal significance'. It was 'an ordinary word of the English language' and 'should be construed in the way ordinary sensible people construe such words. I ask myself what would the ordinary sensible person have said about this patient's condition . . .? In my judgment such a person would have said "Well this fellow is obviously mentally ill."' (W.V.L. (1974) Q.B. 711, 719, C.A.).

One wonders incidentally why Lawton (L. J.) used the term 'mentally ill'; from the tone of his statement 'mad' would have been as appropriate. Indeed, Hoggett slips unwittingly into this by referring to this judgment as the 'man-must-be-mad-test' (Hoggett, 1984, p. 46). From the perspective of an academic lawyer, Hoggett (1984, p. 46) sees Lawton (L. J.)'s judgment as 'denigrating to the patient and to those who have given the matter careful and considered thought in recent decades' and also as a lost opportunity where the courts could have provided a working definition of mental illness, thereby making it likely that statute law would be forced to follow. Whether so or not one can see why Lawton (L. J.)'s definition fails to please the academic lawyer, presumably because it offers so little by way of a recognition of the complexity of the task.

It is all the more strange then that the DHSS definition should have been withdrawn, and for the most curious of reasons (namely that 'a lack of definition has not led to any particular problems', DHSS (1978) para. 1.17). For whom has it not led to any particular problems? Those who operate the Act or those at the receiving end? Generally speaking, definitions or the lack of them are of little consequence and often remain matters of convenience (except, of course, in legal matters). Legal definitions help determine entry into certain types of facilities or determine who shall receive this or that type of punishment. They also exclude those failing to meet the definitional requirements. The need to include and exclude is equally important if rights (and, in this case, the right to treatment) are to be matched with rights to remain free from coercion. As matters now stand, mental illness – the most common form of mental disorder, and the form most often used in compulsory admissions – remains undefined and, in the 1983 Act by implication, therefore a matter solely of clinical judgment.

Turning to 'severe mental impairment' and 'mental impairment', it will be remembered that severe mental impairment is a major form of mental disorder, that is it justifies admission even if hospital treatment is unlikely to do the patient good. 'Severe mental impairment' and 'mental impairment' replaced 'severe subnormality' and 'subnormality' in the 1959 Act, which were defined primarily in cognitive terms. As a result it was said that subnormality and severe subnormality had come to be regarded as pejorative, causing offence and distress. These earlier terms were also criticised as taking no account of social functioning. The DHSS in 1978 suggested they be replaced by 'mental handicap' and 'severe mental handicap' (DHSS, 1978, para. 1.21) but 'mental impairment' and 'severe mental impairment' were preferred eventually. (The differences between the levels of impairment are whether the person is 'severely' impaired or 'significantly' so; a difference almost impossible to determine yet, also to be a matter for clinical judgment.) Whether 'impairment' – in its severe or significant form – will be seen as less pejorative is of course doubtful. Some critics, MIND in particular, see the new terms as producing their own set of prejudices and alienation and rejection, others that the terms imply the patient had been reduced somehow from a hitherto higher level of functioning (quoted in Jones, 1984). Yet it is difficult, perhaps almost impossible, to find other acceptable or suitable terms which are or will themselves remain free of pejorative overtones.

When we look at what constitutes the legal definition of mental or severe mental impairment however, additional problems arise. We are told in the 1983 Act impairment means 'a state of arrested or incomplete development of mind which includes impaired intelligence and social functioning, significant or severe and is associated with abnormally aggressive seriously irresponsible conduct'. Yet 'social functioning' can include matters of taste, based on personal evaluations of various forms of morality. What does 'arrested or incomplete development of mind' mean? What does 'associated with' mean in this context? It was pointed out in the parliamentary debates (11 May 1982) that 'associated with' could be construed as being related to any event that has occurred at any time in the past. The official reply was interesting. The Secretary of state said 'associated with' had the effect of asking people to determine the current state of the patient when deciding whether to detain him. They should be asking whether his state of mind makes him liable to be violent or seriously irresponsible unless a detention order is made. The patient's past conduct, said the Minister 'may be highly relevent as evidence as a way of appraising his current conduct and state of mind'. Even so, it does not meet the criticism that there is a lack of precision in the terminology.

I do not wish to be overly critical here for I recognise there is some merit in the use of the term 'impairment' derived as it is from the International Classifications of Impairment, Disabilities and Handicaps and meaning any loss or abnormality of psychological, physiological or anatomical structure or function (WHO, 1980). There is merit too in insisting that such patients should exhibit qualities which set them off from those currently referred to as mentally handicapped. Parliament's intention was clear: it was to avoid using 'mentally handicapped' in the Act for this would be seen as offensive to those referred to as handicapped elsewhere. Parliament, in response to pressure from the Royal Society for Mentally Handicapped Children and Adults (MENCAP) did not wish to equate mental handicap with mental disorder, or make the terms synonymous in the public mind. Nor did it wish to convey that handicapped people could be detained because of their condition, uncomplicated by other factors. The government was correct therefore in changing handicap to impairment – or, if not then, to use a term other than 'handicap'. The definitions of the new terms remain open to question.

What will be the effect of the 1983 Act on the mentally handicapped? It is expected that those whose condition deteriorates will be reclassified as impaired or severely so and be compulsorily admitted to hospital if necessary. If and when their condition improves, they revert to the original mental handicapped status with all its attendant legal advantages such as priority housing etc. Mental handicap as currently understood is a permanent disability which is detectable from an early age and is often associated with genetic or perinatal damage (Gostin, 1983, p. 3), hence the eagerness to disassociate the mental handicapped from the legislative divisions of mental disorder. As such, the new legal definitions have gone some way to meet that point (parliamentary debates, House of Lords, 1 December 1981). Sadly, however, this is not the end of the matter. Mentally handicapped people originally classified under the 1959 Act as 'subnormal' or 'severely subnormal' have not been re-examined to see if they fall within the new classification. To date (1985) they have all been automatically reclassified as mentally or severely mentally impaired (Gostin, 1984).

The final subdivision of mental disorder, psychopathy, needs little to be said of it, and even less for it. Psychopathy is defined in the 1983 Act as 'a persistent disorder of disability of mind, whether or not including significant impairment of intelligence, which results in abnormally aggressive or seriously irresponsible conduct'. Compare this with the definition of mental impairment and, if there is a distinction to be made, it is so fine as to defy surely the most eminent lawyer or psychiatrist. We need not go over the general criticisms of 'psychopathy' for they are legion except to note that the term has been abandoned in most countries other than in England and Wales and criticised by the World Federation of Mental Health in 1967 as being beyond definition. Yet it is still retained in the 1983 Act, this time on the somewhat lame excuse that to delete it would deny and rule out any possibility of treatment in the future for psychopathic people (DHSS, 1978, p. 8). Seemingly if one has to find something in favour of its inclusion in current legislation then at least psychopathy is classified as one of the minor disorders; also stricter requirements have been imposed for the renewal of detention of patients classified as psychopaths than hitherto.

There remains the generic term 'mental disorder'. This is defined in the Act as 'mental illness, arrested or incomplete development of mind, psychopathic disorder and any other disorder or disability of mind'. Mental disorder is more than that contained in the four subconditions. For example, 'arrested or incomplete development of mind' is wider than that contained in the definitions of psychopathy, mental impairment, severe or otherwise; 'any other disorder or disability of mind' is and was intended as a catch-all phrase. However certain restrictions have been added to place limits on its use; namely that a patient cannot be dealt with as suffering from mental disorder 'by reason only of promiscuity or other immoral conduct, sexual deviancy or dependence on alcohol or drugs'. The 1959 Act contained similar restrictions and they were also included to avoid mental disorder being too closely equated with such types of conduct. The 1983 Act has extended these restrictions to include dependence on alcohol or drugs. Even so, patients dependent on alcohol or drugs can still be detained should they have an accompanying mental disorder, say a mental illness such as depression.

As far as the terms affect the admission procedure, patients can be admitted as suffering from mental disorder rather than one of the more specific subtypes. This is so when they are admitted for assessment, or prior to assessment when they are taken to a place of safety by a police officer. The former under Section 2 of the 1983 Act can however be for 28 days and patients so detained may also be given treatment according to the same rules as those on the longer treatment order. The latter can be detained under Sections 135 or 136 for a maximum period of 72 hours. Patients can also be admitted under Section 4, the 72 hour emergency order, as suffering from mental disorder. It is only under the treatment order, Section 3, that medical practitioners are required to state that the patient suffers from a more specific condition – that is, as under one of those four subcategories. In practice, assessment orders, place of safety orders and emergency orders are by far and away the most common forms of admission (about 14 000 compared to 1700 under treatment orders in 1981), which means that most patients enter hospital under the widest possible diagnostic lable.

One can see how it might be unrealistic to expect police to make a detailed diagnosis when detaining a patient in a place of safety prior to assessment by a qualified medical practitioner, or perhaps a general practitioner or social worker when faced with an emergency. It is surely not an unrealistic expectation to have of a qualified psychiatrist, who may incidentally also deal with emergencies, and is one of two medical practitioners required to decide if the patient requires compulsory admission under Section 2 (this section allows the patient to be detained for up to 28 days). I do not think it is unreasonable in those circumstances to expect a more sophisticated diagnosis than that covered by the term 'mental disorder'.

These then are the major legal categories governing the 1983 Act. Often they are inprecise and sometimes they are obscure, vague or difficult to understand. They allow a great deal of lattitude and, in spite of claims to the contrary, do not I fear advance our understanding greatly. They represent, as I have said before, a lost opportunity. One would hope that future mental health legislation does not repeat this mistake for legislation is often more than a legal document with all its intricasies and claims to protect and preserve rights. It is as often a showpiece, a hallmark to the professions it represents. In this instance the 1983 Act can do little for psychiatry and no more, I fear, for the law.

Finally, it needs to be noted that the 1983 Act uses terminology which is ambiguous. I do not mean by this the legislation is ambiguous for that is sometimes so; rather, I mean that terms like 'The Mental Health Act' are ambiguous for the Act is not about mental health but about ways of controlling mental disorder. To a large extent the official terminology has to be accepted; this is not the place to debate the existence of (say) mental illness or whether mental hospitals are hospitals in the accepted sense of that term. The aim here is more circumspect. Yet I do not wish to convey that the use of such terminology implies its acceptance, merely that the terminology is convenient and avoids entering into detailed arguments not central to the main theme.

Yet why should the 1983 Act be of interest? Consider first what the Act is intended to achieve: it aims to amend the 1959 Mental Health Act without challenging the principles of that earlier legislation, by preserving and strengthening the rights of the patients. Perhaps those principles ought to have been challenged more vigorously, perhaps even thrown aside, but that apparently was not the intention. We may have to wait a decade or so before that happens. Yet the Act remains interesting in itself for it shifts our view of mental disorder to one which no longer assumes the optimism of the 1950s or believes that the right to treatment is absolute. These changes in the legislation in England and Wales are only part of a change worldwide which seeks to reduce the paternalism of an earlier age, to identify the rights of the individual patient, and to reduce (albeit marginally) the power and prestige of the psychiatric experts. Of course not everyone would welcome such changes but, in my view, they represent something of an advance, if only because the new legislation produces doubts where once there was certainty, and shows that there are other ways forward even if those ways sometimes appear unclear.

It is not my intention to speculate on the nature of the social movement which brought about these changes or give a detailed background report to the 1983 Act, for this has been done elsewhere (Bluglass, 1985). Nor is it my intention to approach this piece of legislation with nostalgia for the past, or believe that a few tidying up exercises were needed to return to an earlier harmony. To do so is to cling to a belief that the Mental Health Act of 1959, which implemented the recommendations of the Percy Committee, was as one notable psychiatrist called it 'the most humane and imaginative piece of legislation enacted this century in relation to the mentally ill anywhere in the world' (Roth, 1985). In some respects it was, for it hastened the move towards informal admissions. Yet there was a darker, more sinister side represented by the experiences of many mental patients who suffered at the hands of those whose duty it was to care for them. That is, those patients who were illegally admitted to mental hospitals, who entered hospitals with no right of appeal against their detention, and whose treatment involved permanent damage to brain tissue. The humanity of the 1959 Act was sometimes one-sided.

Those who cling to the nostalgic view have found a new term of abuse, the libertarians. That is people who are seen to be anti-medical in general, anti-psychiatric in particular, and in support of the patient to the exclusion of the patient's family and friends. There may be some libertarians who follow this line, but there are many brands or strands of libertarianism. The abuse tends to be given to anyone who is critical of a form of medical paternalism that once dominated, for – like it or not – psychiatry is now public property, quite different to 20 years or so ago. Moreover, there is emerging a sustained critique of professionals and professionalism and, if that critique is sometimes hostile to the established order, then so be it. Psychiatrists must learn to live with it as have other occupational groups over the years. In these essays I have tried to be critical without being hostile and do so from the perspective of someone who believes that groups with power, and especially power to detain people against their will, must always be subject to scrutiny. If that is libertarianism I am willing to be so classified, although I think other descriptions are more apt.

Section I

The admission of patients to mental hospitals

CHAPTER 2

Social workers and applications

The status and power of the modern social worker have increased greatly over the last 30 years or so. Then as mental welfare officers, and before that as duly authorised officers under the 1890 Lunacy Act, and before that as Poor Law relieving officers they were regarded as lowly beings, occasionally patronised and often misunderstood. Evidence to the Percy Commission illustrates the point.

Chairman. I confess the name (Duly Authorised Officer) puzzles me. For half the time he is a mere transporter, and that is how he is usually thought of. He is duly authorised to transport a mental patient who has been properly certified. On the other hand he has certain independent duties to watch over the safety of the public . . . and the two functions do not fit together.

Medical Officer of Health. He does other things: he prepares the documents. He gets the documents ready on behalf of the relatives in certain cases. I think one feels a little doubtful about it but the only thing one can say is that they do their work well on the whole. They are quite an intelligent crowd of people. They take their work seriously and are seldom if ever complained about.

HMSO (1954–7), Day 4.

This exchange is interesting. On the one hand it provides a useful summary of the duties of social workers under the 1959 Act and, to some extent, under the 1983 Act too; that is as transporter, as protector of the public, as the person who prepares documents (sometimes on behalf of the relatives) and who helps the relatives generally. Yet, on the other hand, it displays a patronising tone unacceptable nowadays. A contemporary Medical Officer of Health would be more respectful of social workers, even if a little irritated by them. He would recognise their increased power and influence and recognise also their enlarged duties in mental health matters

17

although he may be sceptical of their effectiveness. However, under the 1983 Act, social workers have additional duties: to interview the patient and to advise the psychiatrist on alternatives to hospitalisation. In contrast, the powers of the medical profession have if anything been slightly reduced.

There is nonetheless something rather odd about social workers being involved in mental health legislation anyway. Most other countries seem to operate without social workers, the obvious exception being Holland. Some use the police, some relatives, some physicians, some a mixture of all three; in Italy, the Mayor is involved (Sarteschi *et al.*, 1985). Procedures vary too; some countries use the courts, others do not. Yet all seem to require an application prior to admission; that is a non-medical procedural device to bring the psychiatrist to the attention of the patient and to transport the patient to a hospital, if required. That social workers are used in Britain is to some extent a historical accident but, if things were different and there was an opportunity to start afresh, I doubt if there would be great changes. Social workers may not be everyone's favourite occupational group but functionally they provide a service and fill gaps. Even the staunchest critics of social work would not I think suggest they be replaced, although powers and influence of social workers might be regarded as excessive. One must ask, however, who else is there? Relatives or police, perhaps, or some other occupational group specifically trained for the purpose? In practical terms we have to make the best of what is available, and social workers in Britain are best-suited to fill that particular role.

Historically the Poor Law relieving officers had duties to remove patients to a workhouse or public asylum. In this they acted alongside church wardens, constables and officiating clergymen. Under the 1890 Lunacy Act many of these practices continued but, with the break up of the Poor Law and later with the introduction of the National Health Service, the relieving officer came to be called the duly authorised officer. Later the Percy Commission recommended the duly authorised officer be known as the Mental Welfare Officer (see HMSO, 1957, p. 139, note 3). When social work was reorganised under the 1970 Local Authority Social Services Act following the Seebohm Report (HMSO, 1960) the Mental Welfare Officer became the social worker. Under the 1983 Act there is now the Approved Social Worker, that is 'an officer of a local social services authority appointed by this authority for that purpose' (1983 Act, Section 145(1)) i.e. approved by the local authority as being competent to deal with compulsory admissions.

In this sense, the social worker has survived, whereas the clergymen and church warden have not for they no longer have duties in the compulsory admission procedure. The constable has a relatively minor part to play, being largely reduced to dealing with matters under Section 136 (see Chapter 4). To some extent, survival has been by default for the Percy Commission said little about social workers or applications generally. Yet social work fitted easily into that Commission's secular and medical view of mental illness. The more so as the Commission regarded social workers as public officials (HMSO, 1957, para. 402) and it was necessary, said the Commission, to have officials advising relatives on matters relating to compulsory admissions and providing a backup to the medical services. Who better than the social worker to coordinate procedures and transport the patient to the hospital?

Survival has been bought at a price. Demands placed on social workers are greater now, as are expectations, and increasing powers and responsibilities have led to demands for higher levels of competency. Not surprisingly then the 1983 Act tried to raise standards; social workers are to be 'approved' and 'in order to be approved social workers must demonstrate appropriate competence in dealing with persons suffering from mental disorder to their employing authority' (Section 114(2)). It is expected that about 2500 social workers will be so approved, providing an elite group of experts – or a divisive impact on generic social work, depending on how one sees it.

There is and will continue to be a debate on the type of training and the form of assessment for Approved Social Workers; that is whether training should include the wide sweep of the argument linking mental disorder to its social context or whether training should concentrate on assessment of individual patients (see Olsen, 1983). Unhappily these types of questions must be shelved having been replaced by the unseemly squabbling between the National Association of Local Government Officers (NALGO), the trade union to which some social workers belong and the employing authorities. There have been disputes about regrading (that approved social workers be given a higher status than hitherto) and about higher pay for the extra duties and responsibilities. There have been boycotts and demonstrations by some social workers against the Approved Social Work scheme, whilst others (clearly out of touch with union policy) have been expelled from their union for going ahead with examinations. A parliamentary committee (in 1985) described the situation as 'bordering on fiasco' (HMSO, 1985). All of which has further damaged the public image of social work. For, irrespective of the rights and wrongs of the various arguments, there is evidence that some form of training is required. Social workers operating the 1959 Act knew little of the legislation, were often administratively unsound and occasionally appeared to know or care little about the importance of the task in which they were involved (Bean, 1980). Inevitably, the patient suffered. Under the 1983 Act there is at least a recognition that some form of training is required even if, at the time of writing (1985), there is no national programme as such. It will be interesting to see the impact of these training programmes on social work practice as and when they come, and interesting too to see the way in which social workers approach their new task. Yet after these disputes have been settled others will remain, some created by the legislation and others by fellow practitioners (such as those in the medical profession). These, I suggest, are the most intractable.

Social workers, relatives and the application

Approved Social Workers are required to undertake a number of tasks under the 1983 Act, the major one for the purposes to be considered here is to make the application; that is to apply to hospital managers for a patient to be admitted. They share this task with the patient's relatives. Yet why should there be an application at all?

There are, I think, many reasons for an application, some administrative and some not. Those which are not centre around the need to correct a possible or supposed medical zealot who may try to railroad a patient into a mental hospital or act in some other way deemed to be against the patient's best interests. Applications have, I suggest, parallels with consent in general medicine where the patient is asked to agree to an operation or treatment. In effect, the social worker making the application agrees to treatment and detention for and on behalf of the patient, acting presumably in the patient's best interests.

For an application to be effective, it must permit the applicants the freedom to make choices or, as the Percy Commission said, '[the applicants] must be free to accept or reject medical advice and decide whether or not to make the application for admission to hospital' (HMSO, 1957, para. 404). The obvious people to provide that corrective are the patient's relatives who, on the basis of protective kinship, are expected to act on the patient's behalf and make decisions when the patient is unable to make them for himself. Relatives may be unreliable and protective kinship a volatile commodity. For, whilst some relatives may wish to protect patients, others may not – preferring to act for other reasons and in other interests. Some relatives, for reasons best known to themselves, may prefer someone else to act on their behalf. Moreover, there may be instances where there are no relatives or, if there are, they are unavailable, temporarily or otherwise. The social worker's task therefore is to act for and on behalf of the relative where none is available, and against the relative if the relative does not act in the patient's best interests. To quote the Percy Commission again: 'many relatives who accept the need for compulsory admission to hospital would undoubtedly prefer not to have to sign the application themselves . . . a social worker should also be able to make the recommendation when there is no known relatives available . . . and (where necessary) to make the application against the wishes of the relative' (para. 403). The 1983 Act, Section 11(1) says '. . . an application for admission for assessment, an application for admission for treatment and a guardianship application may be made either by the nearest relative of the patient or by an approved social worker; and every such application shall specify the qualification of the applicant to make the application'. The priority of the respective relatives is defined in Section 26(1) and (4) with husband or wife being listed first, then son or daughter, then father and mother and so on.

Note that the 1983 Act says the application may be made by the relative or social worker. Does this, I wonder, indicate a preference? Perhaps not yet, the rights and duties of social workers and relatives in the admission procedure are phrased in such a way as to produce friction between these two groups – the more so as the legal powers granted to social workers and relatives differ (although they are expected to fulfil roughly similar tasks). Consider first the relatives (to be more precise, the nearest relatives but – for convenience – we can simply call them relatives). The 1983 Act gives relatives the right to make an application (under Section 11(1)). The relative also has the right to be informed if the application is to be made by the social worker – this presumably to remedy an earlier anomaly where, under the 1959 Act, the relatives were rarely informed and often discouraged from taking part in any proceedings (Bean, 1980). Also under the 1983 Act (and repeating Section 54(1) of the 1959 Act) the social worker must 'have regard to any wishes expressed by relatives of the patient . . . that it is necessary or proper for the application to be made by him' (Section 13(1)). Quite what this means in practice is difficult to say. However, relatives also have the right to apply to the local social services authority to direct an Approved Social Worker to take the patient's case into consideration and be informed by the social worker if an application is not made (Section 13(4)). These rights are in addition to those which allow the relative to take his case to the general practitioner (GP) for consideration and to proceed by way of the medical rather than the social services. There are also special rights granted to the relative concerning the discharge of detained patients, but not to the social worker (Section 23(2)(a)), and a right to appoint a medical practitioner to examine the patient on the relative's behalf.

In contrast, the social worker has a duty to make the application. There is also a duty to convey or make arrangements for the patient to be conveyed to the hospital after an application is made; no such corresponding duty is placed on the relative. If the relative makes the application the social worker must still interview the patient and provide the hospital managers with a report on the patient's home circumstances (Section 14). If an application is made for admission for treatment or guardianship, the nearest relative must agree. Such consultation and agreement can only be dispensed with 'if in the circumstances . . . it is not practicable or would involve unreasonable delay' (Section 11(4)).

This curious tandem-like quality where relative and social worker have similar but not identical powers inevitably produces ambiguities about the nature of respective roles. For if a social worker refuses to make an application yet the relative wishes to do so, the application can still be made by the nearest relative. This in spite of duties imposed on social workers to prevent undue compulsory admissions and make applications only when they decide admissions are appropriate (DHSS, June (1983*b*), LAC (83)(7)). The social worker has advantages over the relative. Should a relative wish to make the application and the social worker not, the social worker, armed as he is with knowledge of procedures and, of course, of the admission forms, may be tempted to deny the relatives access to these. We may agree with Hoggett (1984, p. 82) when she says to do so would be most improper, for the Act gives the relatives the right to apply, whatever the social worker may think. It is easy, however, to see how this could come about. Would such a situation be open to remedy? Presumably so, although by its nature difficult to establish, for in mental health legislation, such decisions are made away from public scrutiny. If there is no integrity or if procedures are ignored, the chances of an aggrieved party achieving redress are remote.

Certainly the 1983 Act has tried to secure the rights of relatives in matters of consultation and procedure but will this be sufficient? If, past experience is anything to go by relatives may continue to be ignored. Sadly the British Association of Social Workers (BASW) has never disguised its view that relatives are ill-fitted to make decisions on mental health matters (BASW, 1976), discounting the relative's experiences of living with the patient and the detailed knowledge of the patient's behaviour which comes from close personal contact. The BASW's view is that decisions of this nature require professional expertise. Even if this were so, and even if we were to accept the BASW's other point (that relatives may not always stand as protectors of patient's rights) it is difficult to see why relatives should be excluded. More often than not, the decision to admit depends on the capabilities of relatives to live with and cope with their mentally disordered members. This is not a professional matter though it may involve a professional element; the decision is a personal one linked to moral, economic and social questions. A mother may care for and handle a psychotic child better than anyone else, so too may children of demented parents. These groups of patients are by no means atypical or indeed unrepresentative. Of course the BASW does not suggest or expect the social worker to go ahead without discussing matters with the relatives, for that would be bad social work practice but the BASW's views imply a measure of disrespect for the relative's position.

That apart, any existing confusions between social workers and relatives have been made worse by the DHSS's interpretation of the social worker's role. The Act under Section 13(2) states 'before making an application for admission of a patient to a hospital an approved social worker shall interview the patient in a suitable manner and satisfy himself that detention in a hospital is in all the circumstances of the case the most appropriate way of providing the care and medical treatment of which the patient stands in need'. The DHSS has interpreted this rather generously (emphasis added):

Approved social workers should have a wider role than reacting to requests for admissions to hospital, making the necessary arrangements and ensuring compliance with the law. They should have the specialist knowledge and skills to make appropriate decisions in respect of both clients *and their relatives*. . . . Their role is to prevent the necessity for compulsory admissions to hospital as well as make the applications when they decide it is appropriate.   Para. 12, DHSS (1983*a*).

This interpretation moves away from the earlier definition of the social worker as someone who advises the relatives and acts on their behalf, unless that is the relative is seen as acting against the patient's best interests. The DHSS talks of the social worker making 'appropriate decisions in respect of both clients and relatives'. This does three things: first, it confuses and blurs the relative's rights granted in the Act; second, it advances the notion of the professional social worker able to make professional decisions in matters which more often than not lie outside the social worker's training and experience; third, it ignores the fact that the relative can make an application anyway.

What with one thing and another we seem to have produced an increasingly muddled and confusing situation. Yet this could have been avoided. Why not simplify matters and grant relatives and social workers the same rights and duties with additional obligations on behalf of the social worker to inform the relative of his rights, and duties on behalf of the social worker to convey the patient to hospital as before. Under the present system it is likely that the social worker will dominate, further eroding the relative's rights, and perhaps even bringing the law into some disrepute. This is even more likely as the social worker may see himself as further qualified under the Approved Social Worker scheme.

The social work interview

It will be remembered that the 1983 Act says the 'social worker shall interview the patient in a suitable manner and satisfy himself that detention in a hospital is in all the circumstances of the case the most appropriate way of providing the care and medical treatment of which the patient stands in need' (Section 13(2)). The phrase 'a suitable manner' is I think ambiguous. It was introduced for sensible and practical reasons aimed at directing the social worker's attentions to the plight of those who might have difficulties in communicating effectively: for example, the deaf who might need to be interviewed in sign language, or ethnic and non-English speaking minorities who might need an interpreter. There is however a strong possibility that the phrase will be translated into a professional definition where 'suitable' becomes synonomous with 'professional'.

Even so the 1983 Act now requires the social worker to 'satisfy himself that detention in a hospital is in all the circumstances of the case the most appropriate way of providing the care and medical treatment of which the patient stands in need' (notice that this does not apply to the relative). The reference to 'medical treatment' is the critical one for it requires the social worker to comment on matters which may place him in direct competition with the psychiatrist, and on matters about which the social worker is ill-equipped to pronounce. It implies that the social worker ought to comment on diagnosis and treatment and make decisions about the same. It implies also that the social worker would have sufficient knowledge of the nature of hospitalisation and be able to compare this with other forms of treatment and evaluate accordingly. Can this be so?

Consider the social situation of the interviewer. Many commentators, legal and otherwise, writing on the 1983 Act and the compulsory admission procedure create the impression of an orderly routine where patients are interviewed according to a standard set of requirements. Richard Jones for example says the social worker should not make an application and then look for the medical recommendation to support it (Jones, 1984, p. 33). Emergency psychiatry is, however, a more robust affair where patients are interviewed in difficult circumstances, with the occasional threat of violence, and in social situations which sometimes border on the bizarre. Social workers more often than not have to conduct their interviews as and where they can. Sometimes this may mean being a silent partner in a joint interview conducted by a psychiatrist, sometimes being guided and directed by the psychiatrist, and sometimes seeing the patients first whilst waiting for the psychiatrist. There is rarely the opportunity for the quiet reflective approach consistent with the legal view which demands detailed assessment and evaluation. Of itself, this may not be a major obstacle but it remains an important consideration.

There is also the problem of the psychiatrist or general practitioner being unwilling to divulge confidential medical information to a social worker who is an employee of the local authority. To disclose such information would, according to most members of the medical profession, be a breach of confidentiality and harm the doctor/patient relationship. Yet that information may be critical in the psychiatrist's decision to admit. Examples of such cases appear in my own research: one where the patient had a terminal condition and required urgent medical as well as psychiatric treatment, the other where the psychiatrist strongly disapproved of a GP's prescribing practices which he saw as doing the patient harm. The respective social workers were not informed, the psychiatrists saying somewhat tartly it was none of their business (Bean, 1980.) Unless the social worker receives that information, he is unable to make an appropriate decision and will certainly not be in any position to oppose a medical recommendations should he so wish. The social worker therefore, under the new legislation, is being asked to do more than can reasonably be expected of him.

Furthermore, there is the question of the type of information to be collected by the social worker. Is the social worker making a psychiatric diagnosis, albeit at a low level or trying to do something else? Perhaps yes. Certainly the application itself (Form 4B, Reg.4(1)(e)(ii)) requires the social worker to state the type of mental disorder, where appropriate i.e. mental illness, mental impairment, severe mental impairment or psychopathy. (This is not required of the relative, who merely states he applies for the patient to be admitted.) The social worker is required therefore to have some knowledge of psychiatric disease conditions. In addition, according to the Act, the social worker must say that compulsory admission is appropriate; that is he must be aware and knowledgeable of alternatives. He must also be a referral agent where necessary. The interview therefore must be aimed at matching the patient's condition with some alternative accommodation whether it be hostel, local authority home or whatever.

In this sense the social worker acts as a diagnostician, or is expected to do so, according to the 1983 Act. Yet, as was said above, the social worker acts as a diagnostician working at some disadvantage. It becomes all the more important therefore that social workers become clear about the aims of their interviews and the methods to be employed. Sadly little attention was given to this in the past, where social workers operating the 1959 Act had only a hazy knowledge of their duties and aims (Bean, 1980). Sadly too their professional association, the BASW, in its policy paper prepared in response to the Government's 1976 White Paper 'Review of the Mental Health Act 1959' failed to provide sufficient direction. It suggested the social worker should concentrate on the social situation of the patient and should:

(a)   investigate the client's social situation and how that has developed; and estimate in consultation with others involved the extent to which the social and environmental pressures have contributed to the clients observed behaviour;

(b)   apply professional skill to help modify any contributory personal relationships or emotional factors;

(c)   mobilise the resources of the health service, the community services and acknowledge and use the community as a therapeutic resource;

(d)   ensure that any intervention is the least restrictive necessary in the circumstances;

(e)   ensure strict compliance with the law.   Quoted in MIND (1983).

The proposals of the BASW unfortunately do not meet the basic problem. The legislation does not require the social worker to 'investigate the clients social situation' or 'apply professional skill to help modify any contributory personal relationships'. It requires the social worker to state one of the four types of mental disorders in the case of an application for admission to treatment, and in all others to 'satisfy himself that detention in a hospital is the most appropriate way of providing care and medical treatment of which the patient stands in need.' Moreover BASW's proposals fail to recognise that the scope of the interview is often restricted by the psychiatric condition of the client; florridly psychotic people do not require an examination of the social and environmental pressures that have contributed to their observed behaviour. That is, they do not require it at that time (though it may be useful later, eg. in providing assistance on discharge). Neither is there time nor the opportunity to 'apply professional skill to help modify any contributory personal relationship or environmental factors'; again this is not relevant to the task in hand. It may help the client's social relations later but that is not the purpose at the time of the interview.

Furthermore the BASW's proposals also ask too much of the social worker. To require the social worker to 'mobilise the resources of the health service, the community services and acknowledge and use the community as a therapeutic resource', as well as to 'ensure that any intervention is the least restrictive necessary in the circumstances' is to ask him to be familiar with more than can be reasonably expected. It would require him to know the community resources, which in a large city would be varied and probably change daily, and to be familiar with a range of resources defined and accepted as less restrictive than a hospital. It is an almost impossible task. More than that it is not necessary, unless social work is prepared to take onto itself obligations over and above that required by the legislation.

There are similar unrealistic expectations in the proposal by Rolf Olsen entitled 'A curriculum for the training and assessment of the Approved Social Worker' (Olsen, 1983). He wants

to develop a model of crisis intervention which emphasises the interaction between people and the systems with which they have contact, and which stresses the need to consider the personal, social and physical needs of the individual and his living group. It should take account of the individual's right to privacy independence and the exercise of choice; the importance of collaboration and establishing 'contracts' which clarify needs, goals and the strategies to achieve them; a treatment or helping focus which is concerned not only with alleviating the problem but also with total functioning and enrichment; the importance of inter-professional cooperation and endeavour. Olsen (1983) p. 11.

One may applaud Rolf Olsen's optimism and enthusiasm but doubt if such ambitions could ever be achieved, let alone under the syllabus for the course which he later provides lasting for 13 days! Again, the emphasis like that in BASW's proposal is all wrong; it asks too much of the social worker and moves too far from the legal demands imposed on him. The social worker interview as defined by law, (or at least according to my interpretation of that law) has to concentrate on relatively narrow issues restricted to specific questions; that is, does the patient require compulsory hospitalisation? If not, what are the alternatives? Social workers have no legal voice in the treatment of the patient whilst in hospital, or in the decision as to whether the patient should be discharged. Emergency psychiatric interviews are not like interviews for, say, child care where the reception interview forms the basis of future assessment and treatment. They are not about establishing a 'relationship' providing insights or whatever, nor about assisting the patient to come to terms with his condition (though the relatives may be assisted in this). They are about making a specific decision at a specific point in time. The social worker's skill lies in answering these basic questions and advising accordingly. As I said earlier, it is regretted that the legislation asks more than can realistically be achieved, although less than some others (eg. the proposals from BASW and from Rolf Olsen), and regretted too that the nature of the social work interview produces its own sets of limitations.

Social workers and the medical profession

Social workers work closely with two groups from the medical profession, GPs and psychiatrists, when making the application. With each there is an uneasy relationship, although for different reasons. That relationship with the GP is the most interesting, although often the least productive. The GP, as a member of the medical profession, sees social work from the perspective of a professional who lacks the expertise of the hospital consultant but who nonetheless claim generalist knowledge. As mental illness falls within the medical ambit, the GP claims professional competence in this matter. Moreover generalist medical knowledge is valued in the 1983 Act (Section 4(3)), that is a medical recommendation should be made, if practicable, by a practitioner who has previous acquaintance with the patient. To the GP, the social worker is not a professional, lacking both training and competency. Yet, to the amazement of many GPs, the social worker seems to advance, politically and socially, at a faster pace than the GP.

The social worker views the GP with similar distrust. The GP, obviously not of the calibre of a medical consultant, is seen as dealing with medical trivia (being, at best, a referral agent for the hospital specialist). In mental health matters, the GP has limited formal training or expertise yet claims professional superiority. The social worker sees himself as having more knowledge of psychiatric matters, knowing more of the psychiatric services, and having more experience in dealing with behavioural problems. So, the battle lines are drawn.

Regrettably those descriptions given above are not hyperbolic but represent statements given time and again by social workers and GPs during my earlier research (Bean, 1980). Indeed the pettiness often meant that the patient was adversely affected by these unseemly squabbles. Behind it all there was, I suspect, something larger lurking, something more important: perhaps even competition for power and status. For, taken at face value, the complaints from both sides were reasonable enough: the GPs complained of a lack of professional deportment from the social workers, who in turn complained of exaggerated self importance in the GPs. The intensity of the hostility suggests something more forceful. It relates, I think, to the claims of each group to control the compulsory admission procedure. Indeed, the social work literature and the medical literature contains many such complaints, even if couched in less powerful terms than that given above. Social workers, although perhaps not entirely blameless, have to react to and work with such competition.

Relationships with psychiatrists, particularly consultants, are usually more certain perhaps because the psychiatrist sees no competition about professional dominance. Unlike the relationship with the GPs, there can be a frank exchange of views although in truth it must be said the psychiatrist sees himself as the person whose task it is to run the compulsory admission procedure. He is the specialist, has access to the resources of the hospital and (most importantly) sees himself as responsible for treatment and care. The social worker has, according to the psychiatrist, a secondary role: at best advisory and at worst similar to the position of the relatives. The psychiatrist, as a specialist in psychiatric diagnosis, also claims clinical responsibility for the patients.

What then can the social worker offer? Certainly little in terms of the minutae of psychiatric diagnosis but perhaps rather more in matters relating to assessment of patients within the community setting. At least, that is how the Act sees it. Even there opportunities for manoeuvering are limited, for the psychiatrist can always claim the patient suffers from a disorder (perhaps a physical one) which lies outside the social worker's experience and range. Yet the social worker may not be without influence entirely if the aims and objectives are realistic. Any social worker who begins with the assumption that compulsory admissions are a moral outrage, or who asserts idiosyncractic claims will be less than successful. The social worker who is pragmatic may find his influence greater. If so, he will need to accept that some patients require compulsory admission and begin from there. One feature of success, if that is the right term to use, would be to help transfer some patients to a less restrictive status.

Strangely enough, the Act says little about this. Yet to seek informal admission rather than a formal one or an outpatient status, rather than an informal admission has much to commend it. Of course, even then, there are difficulties. Some patients may accept that they need admission to a mental hospital but change their minds prior to or just after entry. Some psychiatrists will therefore, even if the patient agrees, insist on a formal order knowing from past experience that certain patients are likely to be volatile. The social worker can do little about that.

Apart from that, we can see the social worker's influence operating in the following way. Assume the psychiatrist can make three decisions: one, to propose a formal admission; two, to propose an informal one; and three, to decide against admission yet perhaps to offer outpatient treatment. Most patients will fit readily into their allotted group. That is, there will be some who would always be compulsorily admitted according to the accepted canons of current psychiatric practice; some will be voluntarily admitted for the same reason and some will be offered outpatient treatment. There will be few opportunities for the social worker to negotiate on behalf of most of these patients. In the compulsory group, however, there may be some patients (perhaps a small number) whose status could be regarded as less firm, where negotiations can take place which if successful would transfer the patient to the voluntary category. Similarly in the second group, there may be those who can be transferred to the outpatient group. In this way the social worker may shift the patient's status without clashing head-on with the psychiatrist and may avoid being accused of acting irresponsibly, or avoid accusations of claiming levels of expertise greater than he has. Of course this means accepting the superiority of the psychiatrist's position and comprising thereto. Yet, to operate in such a manner is to provide the 'least restrictive alternative' and, I would suggest, do so within the spirit of the 1983 Act. It avoids, too, acrimonious debates which help no one (least of all the patient) and it offers a genuine negotiating position. This is I think the most that can be achieved in the circumstances, assuming of course that the social worker believes that in so doing he is acting in the patient's best interests.

The social work setting

In spite of what was said above it is curious that the Mental Health Act has been interpreted by social workers as imposing a duty on them of protecting the patient's rights. Why not, for example, the psychiatrist or of the GP, especially when – for instance – Section 3 of the Act requires doctors to address themselves specifically to the least restrictive alternative. What are those rights, and who is likely to take them away? The modern view, claimed by social workers and supported by the current legislation is that the patient has more to fear from the psychiatrist and GP than from the social worker. That being so, there exists a tendency to see the social worker in opposition to the psychiatrist, the latter cast in the role of the less-than-benign doctor 'railroading' patients into hospital against the wishes and best interests of the patient. The social worker then appears, as if by some legal magic, to force the psychiatrist to desist. Is this a realistic picture?

From my experience the opposite could be as true: that is the psychiatrist prevents the patients being railroaded into hospital against the wishes of the social worker and relative. No psychiatrist worth speaking of wishes to fill his hospital with patients who do not need to be there, and to treat people who do not need treatment. That would not be in his or in the hospital's interest. Similarly, psychiatrists do not go around searching for patients, trying to pursuade others to make the application. The psychiatrist has patients referred to him normally from GPs but, just as often, from social workers and relatives. To refer is to ask for advice which may, by implication, suggest that the patient needs medical/psychiatric treatment. From my research (Bean, 1980) about 38% of all such referrals were not admitted, voluntarily or compulsorily. It was the psychiatrist who was keeping patients out, the social worker and relatives who were, more often than not, asking for them to be admitted. We hear often of those cases where the social worker defied medical opinion and prevented patients from being admitted, and this is probably all to the good, but we hear less often of situations where the reverse occurs. Of course it is entirely right and proper that someone should restrain medical zealots, but it is also right and proper that social work zealots should equally be restrained. It is I suppose part of the way we view compulsory psychiatry that those with the greatest power should have the largest number of checks placed on that power, but it is also true that those with the least power must be restrained too.

For this and other reasons, social work fits uneasily into modern mental health legislation. The ambiguities in the nature of the application and the interview are testimony to that. The relationship between social workers and relatives, and between social workers and the medical profession add further tensions. The Act also places duties on social workers which they often find difficult to reconcile. The social worker is protector of the patient's rights during the admission interview, yet protector of the patient's welfare under Section 135 (that is where the social worker applies for a warrant to search for and remove patients who are being ill-treated, neglected or kept otherwise than under proper control). Under Section 137 the social worker has all the powers of a constable when conveying a patient to hospital. And, under Section 138, he has powers to retake a patient who escapes and was deemed to be detained under compulsory detention procedures. The social worker is at the same time protector, friend, prosecutor and constable.

It is of course true that other occupational groups have competing role demands placed upon them; the police, for example, are expected to police benignly. They must be protector and friend one minute and prosecutor and foe the next. So too do lawyers, accountants, doctors etc., for no profession can be so one-sided in its outlook as to avoid contradictory demands. Social work is in this sense unexceptional. But social work training tends to foster the image that the social worker's duty is always to the client who must be protected against all else. Yet, as was said earlier, the Act places a duty on the social worker to act as prosecutor on some occasions and protector the next. Sometimes I think social workers seem reluctant or ill equipped to take on this role, being happier when they see their client as the victim (whether of circumstances or, of other people). The mentally ill person may be the social worker's client but mental disorder does not help identify victims in that simple way. Some clients are clearly victims of their condition and of their social relationships, but some only of their condition leaving in their wake damaged and unhappy relationships. Mental disorder, by its nature, can often produce autocracy and cruelty. In other areas of social work this conflict is avoided; in child care for example intervention can be justified as being in the long-term best interest of the child, so too in working with the elderly. This is not so with the mentally disordered.

Social workers too sometimes find it difficult to operate the law as it is, rather than as they think it should be. In other words, they find it difficult to make the Benthamite distinction between is and ought. This again is largely due to their training, where they are encouraged, or rather, not actively discouraged from believing that theirs is a task directed towards social change. I suppose it is difficult to accept that Parliament in its wisdom has written the Mental Health Act this way when ideological fervour suggests it should have been otherwise, but that is something social workers must come to terms with. Hopefully the Approved Social Worker training programme will encourage social workers to see things differently. Perhaps those whose fervour is the greatest will be discouraged from applying as will those whose stance is anti-psychiatry and anti-compulsion. I have said elsewhere (Bean, 1986) that social work has a restless morality which is to be encouraged. I would hastily add, however, that it should not be encouraged in matters as important as those in mental health legislation, or as crucial as compulsory hospitalisation, should that restless morality lead to decisions where the client suffers or becomes a means to some (perceived) greater end.

There is however another side to modern social work. Social work is local authority social work, that is the Approved Social Workers in England and Wales are employees of the local authority. In this they must act according to the dictates of that authority. If the local authority has a certain style and an accepted approach to mental health matters, the social worker must follow. In Chapter 5 on guardianship for example, it will be shown that some local authorities have never accepted a guardianship order and this may be irrespective of the wishes of the individual social worker. So too some local authorities are reluctant to be involved in Court of Protection matters. The individual social worker is not able to make independent decisions in this sense. (It is not unheard of, for example, for a social worker who refused to make an application to have the psychiatrist call the Director of Social Services and insist another social worker make the application – and for this request to have been acceded to). Many of the training programmes encourage the belief that the social worker is an independant agent able to make decisions irrespective of his employing authority. Yet the social worker is an agent of local government, controlled by the vagaries of local politics, although increasingly controlled further by central government financial regulations. Local authority social work is bureaucratised in the Weberian sense; the social worker has to work within that bureaucracy. This paradox, of the restless social worker, acting within a Weberian type of bureaucracy is less apparent now than earlier this decade, i.e. before the financial restraints from 1980 onward. The origins, nature of and extent of the paradox go far beyond the scope of this chapter, yet it means that the individual social worker can often be blamed for the shortcomings of his employers and employers for the shortcomings of their social workers.

Demands placed on the social worker in mental health legislation are one-sided, by that I mean the social worker is involved in the diagnostic process but not in the treatment. There is no follow-up and no information on outcome. The social worker's task is to help decide whether to commit the patient to an institution which, as far as he is concerned, is the end of the matter. His interest in the patient is transitory lacking the personal contact which is at the centre of his training. He may know of the family, he may even know the patient but (having completed the admission) matters end there. This is not always true, of course. Many patients seen on an emergency basis are not admitted, about 38% (see Bean, 1980) and, should the psychiatrist decide not to admit, it is left to the social worker to care for the patient and his family. Sometimes these patients are disruptive and dangerous. The psychiatrist may have refused admission for this or his own administrative and personal reasons which have rather less to do with matters psychiatric. The social worker cannot easily abdicate responsibility; he is a generalist expected to deal with general social problems.

This form of institutionalised conflict with the medical profession makes the social worker vulnerable. The Act encourages this, as does the DHSS when it says the social worker must 'assess the available options . . . and inform himself as to the availability and suitability of other means of giving the patient care and medical treatment . . .' (DHSS, 1983*a*, para. 38). The medical profession has the authority of rank and of knowledge, the social worker in contrast is a lowly professional. If the social worker rejects medical opinion, on grounds which may be entirely reasonable, the medical practitioner can always ask the relatives to make the application. If the social worker opposes admission and the patient harms himself, the psychiatrist can always say the social worker acted against medical advice.

As in all such matters we take less notice of cases where the social worker successfully prevents an unnecessary hospitalisation; we hear only when things go wrong. The social worker is thus caught in an unenviable position. If the psychiatrist does not admit, the social worker is left with the problem (and the psychiatrist can always say that at the time of the interview the patient did not require treatment); if the social worker rejects medical advice, he can be accused of failing in his duties. It is the price paid by the lowly professional when placed in competition with the expert.

These problems cannot be resolved under existing legislation and, if anything, the 1983 Act has made matters worse. Granting as it does a duty to act against the medical profession it has provided the social worker with little except a certificate of approval based on a course of study which compares unfavourably with psychiatric training. The social worker may claim superior expertise to the GP but the psychiatrist still retains the authority of a superior professional with accesss to the resources of the modern mental hospital. To require the social worker to compete is to ask too much and provide him with too little.

There are short-term and long-term solutions but none which will satisfy social workers for they involve compromises in favour of the psychiatrists. To some extent social workers have not helped their case when, as occasionally in the past they have adopted ideological positions which are deemed unacceptable to psychiatrist and patients alike. If the social worker is to be seen as a professional worthy of consideration he must compete on the basis of professional expectations. These expectations involve demonstrating that he has certain skills as well as a thorough knowledge of the legislation. Hopefully the Approved Social Workers will have that knowledge, for it was certainly lacking hitherto (see Bean, 1980). Short-term solutions mean therefore giving up some favoured ideological luxuries.

In the long-term, the social worker's position will be related to the accepted view of mental disorders, and the facilities outside the hospital. If, as seems likely, mental disorder becomes cast more and more in materialist terms, social workers will have a decreasing role to play. Conversely, if social influences are viewed as more important so too will social work. If mental hospitals continue to close and chronic patients continue to be deposited in the community, leaving the acute to be treated by psychiatrists in general hospitals, social work will be called upon to service the chronic and have little contact with the acute. Yet that is for the future: in the meantime social work must accommodate to the contradictions and limitations imposed upon it under existing legislation.

CHAPTER 3

Medical recommendations and compulsory admissions

All societies requiring patients to be admitted to mental hospitals, whether the admissions be compulsory or not have in some way and at some time to devise procedures whereby qualified medical personnel make key decisions. It was not always so (see Scull, 1979) but the modern conception of mental disorder (or lunacy or insanity, call it what you will) has seen fit to view mental disorder as the province of medicine. The Royal Commission preceding the 1959 Act put it this way, 'Disorders of the mind are illnesses which need medical treatment' (HMSO, 1957, para. 5) We have tended to accept that view – not always uncritically and not always with good grace, I would add, and sometimes with a sort of sullen resignation but generally speaking without rancour. There may be debates about the quality of the medical recommendations, about the form they should take, about the timing of the medical recommendations (that is whether they should precede or follow admission), but the medical recommendations remain the cornerstone of the admission procedure.

There may also be debates about the numbers and qualifications of those who should be involved. That is, whether there should be more than one person making the medical recommendation and, if so, whether the recommendations should be made as a result of a single or joint interview. Should the medical personnel be qualified in psychiatry and, if so, at what level? Is any person qualified in medicine sufficient? The permutations and possibilities are extensive, as can be seen by a comparative survey of existing legislation (see Curran & Harding, 1978, especially pp. 87–94). Often the range of possibilities is affected by the extension of psychiatric facilities; Third World countries, for example, having less complex systems.

35

Possibilities are affected too by the manner in which mental patients are given priority in a health care system and sometimes, it seems, by the level of respect for human rights. There is also the historical dimension to consider; in England and Wales the pauper lunatics detained under the Poor Law were subject to one medical recommendation, private patients (being more influential) had two.

The 1983 Act makes no changes in terms of the numbers or qualifications of those entitled to make recommendations. Nor does it affect the general proposition established in the 1959 Act that mentally disordered patients should be admitted to mental hospital on the same basis as patients admitted to other hospitals. The voluntary mental patient, or the informal one as he is now called, is governed by Section 131(1) of the 1983 Act.

The nature of the medical recommendations

The 1983 Act requires medical practitioners to examine the patient even if the patient is well known to the medical practitioner, for recommendations should not be signed without a prior examination. There are also requirements relating to who should or should not make the recommendation; for example, if the patient is admitted as a private patient, to either an NHS hospital or to a mental nursing home, recommendations shall not come from medical practitioners on the staff of those private institutions. Medical recommendations shall not be signed by the applicant, partners in the same medical practice, husband, wife, father, mother-in-law, daughter and so on (Section 12). Moreover, when two medical recommendations are required (as they are under certain sections of the Act) and the interviews are undertaken separately, not more than 5 clear days may elapse between them; this is all too generous in my view. Nonetheless, these restrictions are intended to prevent collusion between the various participants in the procedure and are, on the face of it, obviously of value – provided they are all kept or adhered to. (Who is to know when they have been violated?) Patients rarely know the law. In these and in other related matters, the honesty and integrity of the rule enforcers have to be accepted. In my own research, many patients were admitted compulsorily against the rules or against the spirit of the legislation; none knew this had taken place (Bean, 1980).

There are three major sections in the 1983 Act concerned with the compulsory detention for non-offender patients. At the risk of being legally tedious the grounds are as follows.

(a)   Section 2, the 28 day assessment order. The grounds are
         (i) The patient is suffering from a mental disorder of a nature or degree

which warrants the detention of the patient in a hospital for assessment (or for assessment followed by medical treatment) for at least a limited period, and

(ii) that he ought to be so detained in the interests of his own health or safety or with a view to the protection of other persons.

(b)   Section 3, the 6 months treatment order. The grounds are

(i) The patient is suffering from mental illness, severe mental impairment, psychopathic disorder or mental impairment of a nature or degree that makes it appropriate for him to receive medical treatment in hospital, and

(ii) in the case of psychopathic disorder or mental impairment that such treatment is likely to alleviate or prevent a deterioration of his condition, and

(iii) that it is necessary for the health or safety of other persons that he should receive treatment, and that it cannot be provided unless he is detained under this section.

(c)   Section 4, the 72 hour emergency order. The grounds are it is of urgent necessity for the patient to be admitted and detained in hospital under section 4 of the act, and for the reasons given under section 2.

Notice that in Sections 2 and 4, the grounds are mental disorder (i.e. the generic term) but in Section 3 one of the four types of mental disorder needs to be specified and that in the case of psychopathic disorder or mental impairment 'such treatment is likely to alleviate or prevent a deterioration' in the patient's condition. Also, in Section 3, the grounds require the medical practitioner to state that treatment cannot be provided unless the patient is so detained. For the purposes of this discussion we can take Sections 2 and 4 as ideal types and reduce the grounds to the simpler statements that the medical recommendations involve a decision about the mental disorder plus that of the patient's health, safety or the protection of others. In the latter, the patient's health and safety derives from the ancient concept of *parens patriae*, literally the state as father and protector of the people, and the protection of others from ancient police powers. (see also Bean, 1985).

Consider the question of the mental disorder. The Act says it must be of a nature or degree which warrants the detention of the patient in a hospital; that is the patient cannot be detained under this section because an assessment is required or for some similar matter requiring consideration. The medical practitioner decides on the basis of a clinical evaluation of the patient and recommends detention if the psychiatric condition 'is of a nature or degree . . .'. For these purposes, matters relating to the likelihood of the patients harming himself or others are dealt with later.

The first, and indeed major point, is that we seem to have accepted a number of assumptions which lie behind this piece of legislation. For why should the nature or degree of a mental disorder justify or warrant detention, and by 'nature and degree' I take the law to mean something akin to the severity of the psychiatric condition. We do not detain patients suffering from other medical conditions if they have a more serious condition than hitherto. Are mental patients qualitatively different then? The Percy Commission thought they were, as the following statement shows: 'if the patient himself is unwilling to receive the form of care which is considered necessary there is at least a strong likelihood that his unwillingness is due to the lack of appreciation of his own condition deriving from the mental disorder itself' (para 317). Mental disorders then set the patient apart; the patient's inability to appreciate his condition is due to the mental disorder and (being unable to make a decision for himself) detention is justified.

According to the Percy Commission should that disorder be 'of a nature or degree . . .' the patient becomes additionally vulnerable and less able to make decisions for himself.

We can leave unchallenged one related assumption bound up with the patient's unwillingness to be involved in treatment due to the lack of appreciation of his condition. This is dealt with in Chapter 8 on consent to treatment. Rather, I wish to concentrate on some of the other moral implications involved in accepting the Percy Commission's view: a view which has coloured much of our thinking and formed the basis of much current debate on compulsory admissions. Consider it this way: assume a severely demented patient, where the nature of the dementia produces an inability to understand that condition and the degree of dementia adds to that. According to the Percy Commission, that patient would be suffering from a mental disorder of a nature or degree which would require detention. And so, under the Percy Commission's guidelines, detention would be justified. Yet it seems to me that the mental disorder of itself provides no justification for compulsory admission any more than justification exists to detain a patient suffering from appendicitis. A patient, any patient that is, may be grateful that his malfunctioning appendix has been removed but no one seriously suggests the operation be conducted by force. Illnesses may justify treatment, severe illnesses may justify urgent and perhaps specialist treatment but of themselves do not justify compulsory treatments. Mental disorders, and particularly mental illnesses, if they are to be classified as illnesses, must be judged likewise. Of course if they are not illnesses, then the matter is altogether different; in this case, the whole paraphernalia of medicine (and the medical recommendations that go with it) ceases to be appropriate.

The strong impression, or rather the requirement created by the legislation, is that less severe forms of mental disorder do not warrant detention whereas others justifiably do. So at a certain point on a severity scale, to be determined by clinical judgments, the patient can be admitted compulsorily.[1] Yet it is here that moral questions begin to intrude. These may have less to do with the severity of the disorder as such and more to do with the nature of compulsion. For the psychiatrist must first show that detention is morally justified; he must give reasons which makes it more moral to accept the patient in hospital than to leave him where he is. One could of course ask what moral justifications would there be? In the example given above of the demented patient one could say, I suppose, that it is not so much the mental disorder which prevents the patient from making decisions, rather that patients with severe disorders are liable to make the wrong decisions. In which case, detention is justified on the basis of whether decisions are right or wrong. One could say that severe mental disorders impose greater psychological suffering than mild disorders and that of itself provides sufficient justification. If so, then we return again to the question of the patient with his malfunctioning appendix and ask why such severe conditions do not justify compulsory detention generally. Perhaps one would resort to a more open-ended moral argument where the moral justification to detain and prevent suffering is outweighed by all other considerations, and that paternalism is itself morally and self-evidently justified. The oft-quoted comment that the patient will offer thanks when restored to full health is an example of such a view.

Whatever the reasons, and I confess to be unable to find satisfactory ones, it is easy to slip into one of two forms of argument, both of which seem full of errors. The first is that definitively mental disorders produce lopsided or wrong decisions for that is the nature of mental disorders. Unhappily this restates the Percy Commission's argument in a slightly different form. Were this to be so, it of course fails to meet the point that the severity of disorders fail to justify detention elsewhere. The second is that mental disorders justify detention only when linked to the second part of the legal equation which is that mental disorders are likely to lead to harm to the patient or to others. This is not, however, what the Act says and, as Hoggett (1984) insists, the Act is quite specific on that point. The disorder must be 'of a nature or degree'.

It is not easy to disentangle the legal and moral knots, for they take us back to the nature of mental disorder and its manifestations. The law has sadly provided little guidance, nor (equally sadly) have psychiatrists appeared to want to grapple with such moral questions. We are, I think, entitled to know however why the severity of a disorder justifies compulsory admission and we are equally entitled to know the moral considerations upon which such decisions must be made. For, taken together, this means that medical practitioners must consider matters which have less to do with things psychiatric or medical than is apparent in the legislation. They are indeed involved in a complex moral enterprise where the patient's psychiatric condition may of itself be a consideration but only one in a constellation of moral issues. Of course psychiatrists are not unaware of this. How could they be, when faced with patients unwilling to enter hospital? The legislation provides little help on these questions, conveying the impression that scientific clinical decisions are the determining factors; psychiatry has been content to accept that at face value.

What then of the second part of the legal equation – the patient's own health and safety and the protection of others? Are matters less muddy here? Dealing with health and safety (or, more specifically with health) then as a general point it needs to be said that all diseases must be definitively against a persons health, unchecked ones anyway, for that is what diseases are about. Moreover the phrase 'own health or safety' is sufficiently wide to attract the reasonable criticism that it is capable of almost any interpretation. Even so, the most obvious and glaring shortcoming of current legislation is that it neither specifies the severity nor amount of such behaviour required to justify compulsory detention. To be detained in the interests of one's own health and safety is to protect oneself from the risks, temptations, stresses, decisions, concerns and upsets that beset all of us. Or, in other words, to invoke again a comprehensive form of paternalism. As Hoggett (1984, p. 68) says, once a diagnosis has been made, it is too easy to take for granted that refusal to accept help is the result of that diagnosis rather than of ordinary stubbornness, political or religious convictions or a different approach to the calculation of odds. Gostin (1985) insists that objective criteria should be used as the justification for compulsory admission, or what he calls behaviour based on recent and overt acts. Of itself this takes the argument no further, for it does not specify severity or type of behaviour.

The problem is that some psychiatrists insist mental disorders are, if left untreated, likely to induce self-harm; a view which fits neatly into much commonsense thinking. Moreover, one can see how patients ought not to be left until behavioural criteria show themselves for that, in the long run, may further damage the patient and perhaps lead to longer periods of detention. Apart from this there is also a need to distinguish between self-harm, rationally induced, and that not. Self-harm is not, or should not be a question of whether the patient has this or that set of views, or wishes to take this or that set of risks but that his perception of situations are abnormal in some way, and as a direct consequence of his diseased condition. It needs to be specified which perceptions are likely to induce self-harm. Hoggett (1984, p. 68) says the debate ought to be about the kinds of perception and the kinds of thinking which lead the patient to those views where those views are not the same as other peoples'. Hoggett does not go far enough; it is not that the perceptions are different but that they must be directly attributable to the mental condition and, in turn, directly ensure self-harm. That would seem to me to be one way to justify compulsory detention.

For the other part of the requirement (that is 'the health or safety of others'), matters are slightly different. We have long recognised the distinction between private and public acts, a distinction formulated in classical liberal philosophy, the influence of which is retained in much of our judicial system. Private acts preserve that minimum area of personal freedom necessary for the growth and development of individual personalities, and permit an element of sovereignty over one's mind and body. Private acts cease to be private when they involve harm to others. When they do not they must be permitted. So homosexuality between consenting adults provided an obvious example where classical liberalism influenced the Wolfenden Committee to recommend legalising such activities. The current seat-belt legislation, the requirement for motor cyclists to wear crash helmets reverses the trend somewhat. Many of the principles on which modern criminal law relies preserve that liberal distinction. On this basis 'harm to others' is more generally accepted as a justification for reducing freedoms than 'harm to oneself'.

That being so, once legislation uses terms like 'harm to others' it begins to enter into competition with the criminal law. Critics, such as Hoggett (1984, p. 70), see the requirements of medical recommendations under the 1983 Act as creating a special sort of crime called 'anti-social mental disorder'. Hoggett, and others like her, make the entirely reasonable point that mental health legislation can be used to mop up a type of anti-social behaviour about which we disapprove but which we feel reluctant to call criminal. In this she would find approval from many in the sociological or anti-psychiatry lobby including Thomas Scheff. Thomas Scheff (1964) uses the term 'residual rule breaking', that is behaviour which is found to be distasteful and regarded by most as such; in Scheff's terms this easily becomes the catch-all language of modern mental health legislation. It requires the medical practitioner to adopt the role of policeman to detain those whose behaviour is so offensive. Yet unhappily, according to this view the patient has fewer rights when detained under mental health law, the policeman being subject to more constraints. The policeman can be faced with defendants who can call witnesses, cross-examine, and exercise a right of appeal. It is not necessary to take on board the whole argument to accept the germ of wisdom within those statements.

What then appears on the face of it to be a set of psychiatric criteria turns out to be something more complex involving moral issues of some importance. The law has not yet seen fit to try to unravel these arguments yet, to repeat the point, I think we are entitled to know more than is contained in current legislation. Such questions are the law's business and ought not to have been neatly side-stepped in this way. Curiously enough the Percy Commission appeared to recognise the problem, even if it made no attempt to solve it. It said 'no one disputes that there are some circumstances in which society must in the last resort be able to compel some patients to receive treatment or training in their own interests. . . . and some may need to be protected against exploitation or neglect' (para. 316). In other words a moral and social argument prevails. Sadly all we have in current legislation are phrases such as that the patients psychiatric condition must be 'of a nature or degree. . . .' or that harm to self or others are sufficient to warrant detention. In my view they are quite insufficient.

As I said before, we can search in vain for clarification or assistance in this matter from the psychiatric literature where the preoccupation tends to be of diagnosis, treatment and occasionally fears of intrusion into psychiatric realm by social workers and lawyers. The exercise becomes a collusive one where the law provides powers and the medical profession accepts them uncritically. Whilst it remains important to distinguish between legal and psychiatric criticisms, and that which has been stated earlier is mainly a set of legal criticisms, psychiatric acceptance of the law makes medical practitioners parties to such debates. They become jointly involved, the one explicitly so the other by implication. Curiously enough there was little too in the parliamentary debates to suggest that consideration has also been given to such questions, this not being an area of current concern, Parliament preferring to see medical recommendations as being contained by, and a matter of, medical criteria.

It is currently fashionable to decry social work practice within the mental health legislation and, as shown in the previous chapter, social work practice is not immune from criticism. Medical recommendations, in contrast, are usually seen as being free from the vicissitudes that beset the lesser professional groups. Yet this is not so; both groups have problems created for them by the legislation. And as long as medical practitioners shelter under the image that their's is a matter of medical expertise, the same illusions will be fostered, namely that their's is a scientific exercise divorced from moral considerations.

Admissions and discharges

Compulsory admissions under the 1983 Act require two medical recommendations, one of which must be by a practitioner approved by the Secretary of State (under Section 12) i.e. a psychiatrist and normally a consultant, the other, if practical, should be a registered medical practitioner with knowledge of the patient: usually a GP. In an emergency under the 72 hour order (Section 4) one medical recommendation is required, preferably from a GP, but any registered medical practitioner will suffice. Interviews take place prior to admission and there is no right of appeal against the medical recommendations. Admission for assessment (Section 2) lasts for 28 Days and for treatment it lasts for 6 months, renewable for a further 6 months, and then for periods of 1 year at a time.

Why are two medical recommendations needed? Why is not one sufficient, if the medical practitioner is a psychiatrist, perhaps a consultant? The answer can be traced to historical precedents. Those who framed earlier statutes concerned with private lunatics in the mid- and late nineteenth century formulated practices which have remained with us. The architects of nineteenth century legislation had an ever-present fear that one doctor might be corrupted (the nineteenth century had a low opinion of medical men!) and railroad an unsuspecting patient into a private asylum. Two doctors were required, one to act as a corrective against the other. The Percy Commission preceding the 1959 Act (HMSO, 1957) retained that practice but gave it a modern twist. One doctor it said should be a specialist, the other someone with personal knowledge of the patient. They would then bring to the patient specific areas of expertise: one based on knowledge of psychiatry the other a comparable knowledge of the patient, his background and medical condition. So matters have continued.

Unhappily, at a practical level, there are flaws in this argument. The first is that a psychiatrist, particularly if he is a consultant, is an acknowledged specialist in his field. In the same way that a GP would not disagree with the recommendations of, say, a consultant gynaecologist, so he would not disagree with a consultant psychiatrist. Medicine as a status-conscious occupation allows consultants to have ascribed preeminence, having emerged as superior specialists in their field. GPs in contrast deal with, comparatively speaking, medical trivia. That the Mental Health Act allows GPs the right to advise or correct consultants does not mean GPs expect to exercise that right, or that consultants expect them to do so. GPs may be able to inform on the personal or medical history of the patient but consultants would rarely expect them to do more. Inevitably then the requirements of the admission procedure become subordinate to the structural requirements inherent in the relationship between consultants and general practitioners, the more so as the Act allows the respective doctors to interview together. From my experience, when this happens, the GP becomes the silent partner in the interview offering suggestions but rarely an opinion (Bean, 1980, p. 163). In this sense the psychiatrists run the mental health legislation: the GP may report on the medical history of the patient but his competency is not permitted to extend further.

Secondly, the consultant has the wherewithal to decide on the admission itself (that is, if and when the patient should be admitted). Try as he might, the GP cannot get the patient into hospital if the consultant disagrees. (Technically, admission is by agreement with the hospital managers but, in practice, this means the consultant.) The GP may act only as a negative reference group; that is he can keep the patient out, he cannot decide to let him in. Sometimes he would be unwise to try to do this for, having asked for advice, the GP cannot then easily refuse it. The GP is dependent on the psychiatrist to help manage his patient load for there will always be another time and another patient. In practice, any GP who asks for advice is almost duty bound to accept it. This is not entirely true, of course, but it would be a very determined GP who has prepared to do otherwise (perhaps a foolhardy one). I am suggesting therefore that the structural position of the GP reduces the value of the second doctor to act as a corrective against a consultant psychiatrist. In my view it would be more honest and open to accept that the second doctor, if he is a GP, is given a minor part to play and more honest to accept the consultant as the key figure. As things stand, the belief is sustained that two doctors restrain each other by offering diverse opinions when (in practice) they rarely do.

For the emergency order, any qualified medical practitioner can make the medical recommendations (however inexperienced he may be in psychiatric matters). Of course the hospital must agree to accept the patient, but even so the medical practitioner has extensive powers. The 1959 Act introduced such provisions and followed the recommendations of the Macmillan Commission in 1926. That Commission, like its successor, was intent on forging closer links between psychiatry and medicine generally. 'We are not disposed to recommend any differentiation in this respect. Apart from questions of convenience it would tend to demarcate psychiatry as a thing apart from ordinary medical practice, a position from which it is now being retrieved' (HMSO, 1926). The 1957 Commission accepted its predecessor's recommendation without question, being intent too on implementing a similar principle.

One can see that it may not always be possible to obtain the services of a psychiatrist in an emergency; there is always the ultimate barrier – the hospital may not accept the patient, or if it does, then it may discharge the patient if detention is not considered necessary. In contrast to what will be said in Chapter 6, professional discretion here is to be welcomed; indeed perhaps one of the few areas where it is. Even so, to permit one medical practitioner to make a recommendation which results in the compulsory detention of a patient without having to demonstrate an interest or expertise in the subject matter is still something I find difficult to accept. On this basis of course, the psychiatric nurses' holding power – discussed later in this chapter – is more easily justified, for the nurse has at least achieved some experience in psychiatric matters. Consider too that most compulsory admissions under the 1959 Act were under the emergency order (about 60% in all) although not necessarily, of course, on the recommendation of one medical practitioner who may be a GP or someone of similar standing. It is unfortunate then that the 1983 Act did not amend the emergency provisions by insisting at least that the patient should be seen by a consultant psychiatrist on arrival at the hospital. Yet, when all is said and done, it must be accepted other countries permit similar practices where patients are admitted on one medical examination and by any qualified medical practitioner. It seems to work reasonably well elsewhere although, of itself, that is not a sufficient reason to continue the practice in England and Wales.

The three Sections relating to compulsory detention (Sections 2, 3 and 4) permit patients to be admitted for different lengths of time, for different reasons and different circumstances. There is the 72 hour emergency order, the 28 day assessment and treatment order, and the 6 months treatment order. The law insists that those making the medical recommendations give reasons why a patient was admitted under one Section rather than another. For example, the emergency order is to be selected in cases of urgent necessity, the 28 day order for assessment (yet provision is also granted for treatment), and the 6 month order for treatment alone. In one (the 28 day order) the medical practitioner must state the patient suffers from a mental disorder of a nature or degree which warrants detention and for the treatment order that the patient is suffering from one of the forms of mental disorder which makes it appropriate for him to receive treatment. The decision, as ever, is to be based on clinical judgments.

As in much of the law relating to admissions, the terminology permits the maximum flexibility yet is open to the obvious and repeated criticism that it is capable of wide interpretation. Moreover, patients can be transferred from the less lengthy order to the treatment order, subject of course to certain conditions being fulfilled, so it is possible for a patient to be admitted under an emergency order, transferred to the 28 day order and subsequently transferred to a treatment order. He can drop out of the process after the emergency order is completed, or after the 28 day order depending, presumably, on his response to treatment or to other factors relating to his condition. He could even become a voluntary patient. He can be admitted directly to the treatment order, thereby circumventing the shorter orders or be admitted to a treatment order having been just a voluntary patient. The law permits a number of possibilities.

Such flexibility granted to medical practitioners under existing legislation is regarded by them as a major strength. Mental patients, they say, cannot be governed by tight legal categories. Flexibility allows the medical practitioner to make the refined diagnosis later, after observation and preliminary treatments have taken place. Yet flexible legal terminology can create disadvantages for the patient. In the first place those legal categories are not discrete. A patient is to be admitted under Section 2 (the 28 day order) because his mental disorder warrants detention for assessment, and for Section 3 (the treatment order) where it is appropriate for the patient to receive medical treatment in a hospital. The emergency order is for 'urgent necessity'. Most patients could fall within and be admitted under any one of these categories. Furthermore, terminology as loose as that in the 1983 Act can easily permit clinical decisions to override legal requirements. By this I mean that clinical or indeed social considerations can push legal requirements into second place. Loose, or wide, terminology encourages clinicians to see the law as generous rather than creating the impression that the law's task is to separate patients into defined legal categories.

Consider the emergency order: under the 1959 Act it was used extensively (probably accounting for about 60% of all compulsory admissions). In contrast, the long 12 month treatment order was used more sparingly, with the 28 day order used in about 30% of all cases. In my own research, it was clear that many patients admitted under the emergency order were not emergencies in the strict sense of that term. More often than not the emergency order was used as a convenient way of admitting patients without having to obtain a second medical recommendation. What then distinguished patients on the 28 day order from those on the 12 month treatment order? As far as could be seen the psychiatric history of the patient was the determining factor rather than the current psychiatric condition. Patients with records of previous admissions and, especially so if known to the psychiatrist conducting the emergency interview, were more likely to be placed on a treatment order than others with similar conditions. This was not always the case of course, but the trend was significant.

Given the nature of the legislation one ought not I think to expect things to be otherwise. Under the 1983 Act, the psychiatrist is offered three types of order [the short-term one for emergencies, a medium-term one (lasting 28 days) which can now include treatment, and a longer one (for 6 months) reduced from 12 months by the new Act]. There is no pressure on him to formulate a diagnosis at that stage. There are also provisions in the Act to discharge patients from compulsory orders, if seen to be appropriate. There are no legal precedents to consider, nor is the patient granted a right of appeal prior to admission, although he can appeal to a Mental Health Review tribunal after 14 days of the 28 day order. The Act thus provides a considerable measure of clinical freedom.

If, however, one thinks solely in terms of the period spent under compulsion there are advantages for patients admitted under the emergency order. It will be remembered that there are provisions for patients so admitted to be transferred to the longer order if required. Yet few seem to be so transferred. Similarly, there are provisions for patients under the 28 day order to have their orders discharged if compulsion is no longer needed. Few seem to be so discharged. All this is particularly interesting when one considers that many patients admitted as emergencies may not be so in the strict legal sense of that term. Had they been detained under the longer order they would have spent more time under compulsion, to no apparent ill effect. The psychiatrist who admitted all patients as emergencies (see Bean, 1980) may not have acted according to the law, yet may have acted with the approval of the patient. Incidentally, he like so many others, provided treatment under the emergency order so the patient was not at a disadvantage in that respect.

One may not believe that the period spent under compulsion is the important factor, the compulsory admission itself being more critical (for that is what is recorded on the patients file). Some critics would point to the levels of deprivations and indignities common to all patients in mental hospitals, suggesting that compulsion imposes a comparatively negligible burden. That may well be so, but I wonder sometimes if the lengths of orders offered could not be such as to provide shorter periods for observation and treatment. It is recognised that shorter orders might encourage medical practitioners to use them more frequently, but perhaps not. It is worth further consideration.

Turning now to questions of discharge: provisions exist under the 1983 Act for non-offender patients to apply to a mental health review tribunal (MHRT) when placed on a treatment order. Under the old Act, this applied only to Section 26 patients, but now that treatment is formally permitted under the 28 day order, patients on Section 2 can apply to a MHRT after 14 days. MHRTs are dealt with more fully in Chapter 7. At this stage, I wish to consider one or two questions relating to discharges generally, as they apply to non-offender patients.

The first point to make is that under Section 25(1), which deals with discharges requested by the patient's family, the responsible medical officer can oppose discharge if he thinks the patient is likely to act in a manner dangerous to himself or to other persons. Compare this to the requirement for admission when a patient can be detained for his own health or safety or for the protection of others. It is not entirely clear why the requirements for admission should be less severe than for discharge. A legal oversight perhaps or a deliberate attempt to let out those carrying less risk? Either way it is an odd situation. (One shudders to think what could happen if a patient had not deteriorated yet remained as before, being discharged on the grounds that he was not dangerous but immediately readmitted on the grounds of his own health and safety and for the protection of others. Such are the legal anomalies we must forever live with.)

The second point is more general, relating to the lack of attention given to discharges of patient's orders. Apart from a small number of patients discharged through MHRT procedures, and those through Section 25(1) above, most patients find their orders come to an end and they remain as voluntary patients or are discharged. A smaller number are transferred to lengthier orders, or have existing ones extended. Very few patients on the 72 hour emergency order appear to require additional controls (Bean, 1980), suggesting that once in hospital informal controls, from the patient or others, are sufficient. This again supports the argument that shorter periods under detention are preferable as a general rule (although not entirely, for demented elderly patients have slightly more rights when under detention than as voluntary patients – including their right to consent to treatment; see Chapter 8). That apart, most orders simply come to an end, implying and providing tacit approval for the compulsory admission procedure.

Questions remain. Are patients placed on orders qualitatively better off? What are the criteria for using such orders in the first place? What is the effect on patients of compulsory orders, long-term and short-term? We simply do not know. There does not appear to be much eagerness to find out. The 1983 Act continued the practices provided under earlier legislation, accepting them largely without question and allowing the whole procedure to run along as before. It is strange that this should be a neglected area of research given the large number of patients detained each year. Has it, I wonder, something to do with a reluctance to provide research facilities or that assumptions are made about the way in which medical recommendations always operate to the benefit of the patient? I wonder.

Voluntary patients

Voluntary or informal patients are considered hardly at all in the 1983 Act, except on matters relating to the need to provide facilities for their admission or the detention of such patients wanting to leave hospital against medical advice. In the first Section 131(1) says:

nothing in this act shall be construed as preventing a patient who requires treatment for mental disorder from being admitted to any hospital or mental nursing home in pursuance of arrangements made in that behalf and without any application order or direction rendering him liable to be detained under this act or from remaining in any hospital or nursing home in pursuance of such arrangements after he ceased to be so liable to be detained.

Section 131(2) specifies the age at which a person can be so admitted as an informal patient, namely 16 years. Section 131 retains provisions made in the 1959 Act, whereby informal patients can be admitted to hospital without certification or under any other legal or quasilegal requirements. Informal patients generally have no restrictions on their right to refuse treatment or leave the hospital or nursing home as and when they wish. About 90% of all patients are informal, placing England and Wales at about the top of the international league. It was not always so, for in the late 1930s, and even after the 1930 Mental Treatment Act was passed (designed to admit informal patients), about 90% of patients were still compulsory (see Bean, 1980).

The 1959 Act provided the major impetus to admit informal patients and was successful in this respect. It nonetheless retained some anomalies which the 1983 Act has removed, for example the power to withhold a patient's mail (Section 134) and the removal of foreign or alien patients, which cannot now be undertaken except by reference to a mental health review tribunal. The legal position of informal patients in respect of the right to vote whilst in hospital has been strengthened. Also it remains unlawful for an informal patient to be prevented from leaving hospital if he wishes to do so, whether by direct physical restraint or locking doors or placing the patients in seclusion. Unhappily, some patients are still detained in this way and, from my knowledge of the system, with the tacit agreement of all concerned, including members of the patient's family.

It would be true to say however that the 1983 Act has helped enhance the rights and status of the voluntary patient – that is with one major exception, relating to the detention and holding powers granted in Section 5. This section permits a registered practitioner in charge of the patient, or his nominated deputy, to detain a patient already in hospital if the patient wishes to leave, and it is necessary for the patient's health and safety or for the protection of others that he is detained. Under the 1959 Act there was no provision for a Responsible Medical Officer (RMO) to nominate a deputy and this caused some confusion when the RMO was not available. The 1983 Act tidies up this anomaly, although it still does not define what is meant by a patient. When is a person a patient? When he crosses the hospital threshold as it were, or when he arrives in the ward, or after his first medical examination? These are not simply legal niceties; some patients have been lured into the hospital entrance, been classified as an inpatient and had the holding power imposed (see Bean, 1980).

The 1983 Act however introduces a new power. It provides for nurses of a prescribed class to invoke a holding power for up to 6 hours. During this period, the medical practitioner in charge must then consider whether the full holding power of 72 hours should be made (see Section 5(4)).

Why was this power given to nurses? On the one hand, this new power ends the uncertainty nursing staff have felt about their legal position when restraining informal patients. For, of course, there are occasions when an informal patient requires physical restraint and a decision is required as to whether he should leave hospital or not. One would have thought the simplest thing to do would be to inform the registered medical practitioner, or his nominated deputy, and to allow the normal procedure to be followed. After all, these situations rarely develop without some warning. If they do, common law powers exist to restrain patients anyway. In common law an individual is entitled to apprehend and restrain a person who is mentally disordered and who presents an imminent danger to himself and others. The degree of medical or physical intervention used should be sufficient to bring the emergency to an end (Gostin, 1983, p. 8) Why not then use the common law powers if a situation suddenly develops or call the appropriate registered medical practitioner?

Unfortunately, there are political issues at stake here. For behind that power granted to nurses is an influential trade union demanding more and more status and influence for its members. (The Confederation of Health Service Employees; see COHSE, 1978). It seems entirely reasonable to suggest that clarification of the nurses role is desirable, and that the legal position of nurses requires consideration. This, I fear, is not what the argument is about (or not what it is just about). Demands by nursing staff for greater influence in the hospital generally and about which patients should or should not be admitted and the type of treatment to be given are gathering apace. Already trade union action, or the threat of it has led to one patient taking his case to the European Commission of Human Rights (see also Chapter 10). In this instance, the application concerns the prolonged detention of the applicant in Broadmoor hospital as of 1 March 1979 after he had been found fit for transfer to an ordinary hospital at Oakwood, Kent, and the applicant's attempt to challenge the lawfulness of the authority's refusal to transfer him. The transfer was made impossible by the refusal of the nurses trade union (COHSE) to accept patients held under Section 65 of the 1959 Act on transfer from Broadmoor to ordinary mental hospitals, which (nurses claimed) had not the resources for dealing with such patients (Council of Europe, Ashingdean v. United Kingdom, 12 May 1983). The European Court subsequently dismissed the applicant's case, thereby allowing the union to continue with such claims.

The demands of one Trade Union (COHSE) may not reflect the views of the entire nursing profession, the Royal College of Nursing (having the largest number of members) may be altogether more restrained. Threats of industrial action, even from members of one union, can seriously disrupt and place patients in a vulnerable position. The holding power under the 1983 Act was an obvious attempt to placate Trade Union demands. Why limit it there? Why not include all nurses? What is wrong with the other health service employees such as domestics, gardeners or cleaners? Is this merely a silly question or are we witnessing the thin end of the wedge?

In my view, this particular holding power has created a dangerous precedent. It can do little to increase the respect for psychiatric nurses and may do much harm to them. Granting powers of detention to any occupational group must be a major step. It is bad enough that the medical profession and social workers have powers to detain patients without rights of appeal but these powers, with the exception of those granted to the nominated medical officer in charge of the patient, have to be adjusted to the demands of others; if a doctor wants to make the medical recommendation then the social worker must also make the application. Nurses operate under no such constraints. It is also curious that in the parliamentary debates of the Act, few members appeared to be apprehensive about granting this holding power, more appearing to be concerned with the need to hold rather than the power in the holding. As I see it, the effect is to add another occupational group to those already given powers of detention, without in my view justifying such a group or the powers themselves. For, if only to repeat the point, it would have been sufficient to tidy up existing legislation rather than grant new powers. How informal patients will perceive all this will be a matter of great interest to the nursing profession generally and to mental hospitals in particular.

An overview of medical recommendations

The 1983 Act changed little as far as the medical recommendations are concerned and left a residue of problems. Most centre around the looseness of the legal terminology but others are found in the manner in which psychiatric demands shelter and mask moralities. This is not so much a problem of psychiatry as of law, inherited from the Percy Commission's view that mental disorders are illnesses like any other illness and a desire to place psychiatry within the mainstream of medicine. Even if mental illness were of this order and even if it were possible to show that all mental disorders had a materialistic base, there would still be the effects of that disorder to consider. These remain social and moral questions.

As things stand at present we produce many confusions and promote many ambiguities. Consider the question of harm to self. In England and Wales there are no sanctions against non-mental patients who inflict self-harm, for suicide and attempted suicide has ceased to be a criminal offence since 1961. Yet, according to the Percy Commission, sanctions should be imposed on the mentally disordered if they wish to harm themselves, even if the harm is slight. So, to use a most extreme and perhaps a somewhat hyperbolic situation assume a mental patient who was sufficiently mentally disordered and mildly neglectful of himself. After satisfactorily completing his psychiatric treatment he may then commit serious and perhaps fatal harm to himself. That, although obviously regrettable, would not be the business of the Mental Health Acts, nor of anything else for that matter. Yet it serves to illustrate the murky areas in which mental health legislation moves. Protecting patients against themselves on the basis of their lack of appreciation of their condition, due to the presence of mental disorder produces a tangled web of problems and ambiguities – none of which, I would add, have been resolved by the current legislation.

Moreover to insist as did the Percy Commission that mental disorder accounts for a patient's unwillingness to appreciate his condition, takes away his sense of responsibility and places him at the level of a child. Once seen in this way other steps easily follow; it becomes a simple matter to justify actions which involve taking away hospital patients' day clothes, or checking and examining details of their personal possessions whilst in hospital. What greater justification could there be for intruding into the minutiae of the patient's life than the unchallenged assumption that the mental disorder led to self-neglect or self-harm.

On the question of harm to others, matters are no less complicated (one could add that the distinction between self-harm and harm to others is less than clear, for all self-regarding acts influence others to some degree – however small). Nonetheless, if harm to others is to be retained in the medical recommendations, then it seems reasonable to expect a set of guidelines limiting intervention. It also seems reasonable to demand clarification as to the limits of the law, and the limits of a civil commitment procedure (which operates in like manner to the criminal law but without similar safeguards for the detained). And, if it is as reasonable to ask how far should the law go in this matter, it is also reasonable to ask what are people entitled to be protected against. To leave matters as they stand is to invoke suspicion and the accusation that medicine has overstepped its boundaries yet again.

Surrounding the whole process of the medical recommendation is the superiority of the clinical judgment. When clinical judgments are allowed to dominate, as they do in the medical recommendations, they force us to consider why this should be. This is particularly so as psychiatry itself has not been able to demonstrate the quality of its predictive power or show a succinctness of diagnosis. If a science is to be judged in its ability to make qualitative predictions, then psychiatry falls short. There is a good deal of evidence to suggest that psychiatrists tend to overpredict in matters of harm to self and others, indicating that the variables used are given the wrong weights or they are the wrong variables. Diagnostic categories are unreliable in the research sense of that term and the definitions often vague. Yet why are the powers granted to medical practitioners so wide and the rights of patients so limited?

It cannot be denied that psychiatric powers are linked to the status and powers granted to medical practitioners generally and psychiatry has benefited from this. This relative influence of the medical profession as a pressure group is well known. Unlike other areas of medicine, psychiatry is a difficult subject for the law maker to get to grips with. Psychiatry gets away with it, as it were, because the subject is too difficult to encapsulate in a single legislative framework. It is not so much a mystification process, although to some degree it is; there is also the problem of regulating behaviour as varied as that seen as mental disorder. The criminal law can regulate criminal behaviour more effectively because it relies for the most part on objectively defined acts. Psychiatry deals more with subjective states. That is why those who demand that medical recommendations be based on recent overt acts have been less than successful in their campaign; the idea is right but psychiatry claims to deal with more than acts, recent or otherwise.

Resolution of these problems, or rather a movement towards meeting the criticisms (for such problems can never be resolved as such), would depend: first, on psychiatrists being able to identify the nature of those conditions they call mental disorder; then, to show how these disorders affect the patient's behaviour in terms of self-harm and protection of others; then, to ask how far the law should go in this matter and to ask what people are entitled to be protected against. This would be no easy task, but is long overdue.

CHAPTER 4

Detention of the mentally disordered in the community

Mental health legislation provides elaborate methods for dealing with the mentally disordered in private dwellings, reflecting the emphasis we place on our indoor culture. Yet it has also to deal with those who are in public places. The mechanism for dealing with this group of mentally disordered is, on the face of it, comparatively simple: legislation enpowers a police constable to remove a person from a public place to a place of safety if he considers that the person is suffering from mental disorder and is in immediate need of care or control. The person can be so detained for up to 72 hours. During that time he can be examined by a doctor and interviewed by an Approved Social Worker in order that suitable arrangements be made for his treatment and care. This power completes and tidies up matters: it completes them in the sense that it deals with public places rather than private dwellings and it tidies up matters in that it makes public places safer. Additionally it provides facilities for those in need of care. If it is agreed that such a system is required, and almost everyone does (see Parliamentary Debates 18 October 1982), one would have thought there would have been little or no debate about it.

This is not, however, so. Section 136 of the 1983 Act (it was Section 136 of the 1959 Act also and one of two sections to keep the same numerical position) has attracted a great deal of controversy, often producing a fierce polemic. As it is a comparatively short section in the Act it seems worth quoting in full.

Section 136(1)

> If a constable finds in a place to which the public have access a person who appears to him to be suffering from mental disorder and to be in immediate

55

need of care or control the constable may, if he thinks it necessary to do so in the interests of that person or for the protection of other persons remove that person to a place of safety within the meaning of Section 135 above.

(2)   A person removed to a place of safety under this section may be detained there for a period not exceeding 72 hours for the purpose of enabling him to be examined by a registered medical practitioner and to be interviewed by an approved social worker and for making necessary arrangements for his treatment and care.

This section does not provide for admission to a mental hospital as such, but for detention in a place of safety permitting further decisions to be made. A place of safety may but does not have to be a police station; it could be a hospital (any type of hospital that is within the meaning of the National Health Service Act 1977), a mental nursing home, a residential home for the mentally disordered or any other suitable place where the occupier is willing to receive the patient temporarily (Section 135). For all practical purposes, it means a police station, for very few hospitals will accept patients on the recommendations of a police constable, and there are few 'other suitable places where the occupier is willing to temporarily receive the patient'. This in spite of pleas from various government agencies that the place of safety should be elsewhere.

Lawyers find Section 136 a rich area for debate, leaving for them many loose ends and definitions. Firstly, there is the problem with 'a place to which the public have access'. Does a football ground, car park or railway platform constitute such a place? The answer is yes, apparently, even if those admitted have had to pay admission fees. Lifts, landings and staircases serving a block of flats however are private (see Hoggett, 1984, p. 139). What would happen if, say, a constable intentionally lured a person from the private to the public place and then detained him? Would this act be lawful? Apparently not. Could the policeman then claim protection under Section 139 (the section giving protection for acts done in pursuance of the 1983 Act)? Perhaps not, but no one is sure. Consider what would happen if a policeman did not detain someone about whom Section 136 could apply, and the person died or injured himself or someone else? What would happen then? Apparently nothing, but a coroner would no doubt call attention to this and may blame the constable publicly for not taking action, although the Mental Health Act does not make the constable's duty clear in this respect.

Secondly, there are legal problems relating to the period of detention. For example, how does a person know when he is on a Section 136 order? There is no formal order to be made as such, nor does there appear to be a general right to make a telephone call during the period of detention. What happens if the person is seen by the appropriate professional staff and they say no further action is required. Can the person be kept up to the 72 hours? Indeed, when do the 72 hours begin (at the point where the constable sees the person or at the point of detention)? If a registered medical practitioner or Approved Social Worker does not want the person admitted to hospital, can he be kept in a police station until someone else eventually agrees to admit him? Again, no one seems to know.

Thirdly, what type of order should be made following a Section 136 order, assuming that is admission to a hospital is desirable? Could there be an emergency order for example? Some lawyers would say there could, others that an emergency has already existed once the person was found in a public place. That is, the emergency ended when the patient was taken to a place of safety, and there can be no second emergency. Those arguing otherwise accept that an emergency existed but say that Section 136 has not resolved matters, simply that the patient has been detained for others to proceed accordingly.

Finally, on a related issue, there has been considerable debate about the length of time the person is permitted to be detained. There is no legal issue here although, for completeness' sake, there are a number of other questions to be raised. The 1983 Act specifies a period not exceeding 72 hours, as indeed did the 1959 Act. Most critics however argue that 72 hours is too long. Some have suggested as little as 4 hours [that from the British Medical Association, BMA (Parliamentary Debates, 18 October 1982, p. 91)], some 6 hours, some 12 hours and some 24 hours (the latter from MIND). The argument to reduce the period of detention seems overwhelming: it does not take 72 hours to get a registered medical practitioner and Approved Social Worker to see a patient. If it does, something is sadly wrong with the service provision. Yet the government remained unmoved during the parliamentary debates on the 1983 Act, arguing that 72 hours should be the maximum period of permitted detention although it expected the maximum to be used infrequently. If a period of 72 hours exists, even if rarely used, there remain opportunities for abuse, or rather opportunities to adopt a somewhat carefree attitude towards the detained person. Or, as one Member of Parliament (MP) put it 'I want to instil a sense of urgency in the matter' (Parliamentary Debates, 18 October 1982). In my view, he was entirely correct, 72 hours is far too long. The BMAs proposal that it should be 4 hours is more acceptable.

The variable nature of the manner in which section 136 of the Act is applied

The official figures show that 1855 patients in England were recorded in 1982 as having been detained under Section 136. (The Mental Health

Inquiry for England in 1977 showed 1494.) A closer look at these figures shows two things: first, that the numbers of patients detained under Section 136 is increasing, this at a time when compulsory admissions generally are decreasing; second, that the use of Section 136 is almost confined to the Metropolitan District in London.

One should, however, be careful of reading too much into these figures or imputing unfairness or whatever. The use of Section 136 may well be unfair in that it appears to be restricted to the London area but unfairness cannot be inferred from these data. To begin with, the figures show only the formal use of Section 136; that is, when the patient was formally detained and a Section 136 form was completed with the patient being seen by the appropriate persons before being removed to a hospital. The point was made during the parliamentary debate (18 October 1982, p. 92) that a more appropriate set of figures would show the numbers detained by the police before being seen by the registered medical practitioner or Approved Social Worker. Currently there is no way of knowing how many patients were detained and subsequently released. Nor do the figures show how many patients were seen yet admitted under other compulsory powers of the Mental Health Act. Nor do we know how many were seen yet charged with a criminal offence, rather than becoming inpatients in a hospital. For, if the police were so inclined, they could find almost any behaviour of an abnormal kind in a public place to be the basis of some sort of criminal charge (Walker & McCabe, 1973). Crime or disease: the police choose.

Moreover, the use of Section 136 (officially, that is), may be entirely dependent on the arrangements made between police and psychiatrists locally and these arrangements mask and distort the true position. It is often difficult to believe that a country as small as England and Wales, with a high density and relatively homogeneous population should have such wide variations in practice. One can, however, no more talk of a national policy here than in say Canada, Australia, the USA or elsewhere. In the Nottingham area, for example, police and psychiatrists had an arrangement whereby psychiatrists were called to the police station to interview detained persons. If the psychiatrist wished to admit the person under compulsory powers, a social worker was then informed. If the psychiatrist did not want to admit the person, he was released, or perhaps charged with an offence, usually a minor one. ['Is he yours or ours?' said one police officer, see Bean (1980).] Under this arrangement, Section 136 was used – but not in the manner prescribed by legislation. No patient was officially recorded as being detained yet, in all other respects, Section 136 was used in the manner legally prescribed. In order to understand the official figures then one must also understand the nature of the arrangements between police and psychiatrists at the local level. To do otherwise is to fall into that well-baited trap which criminologists have warned exists elsewhere in the interpretation of other (official) figures.

Whilst it may be wrong in the strictest legal sense that these informal arrangements exist, they provide flexibility in the system and allow adaptations to be made to local conditions. Without defending these informal arrangements, as far as could be seen they worked quite well. Patients were seen quickly and efficiently by psychiatrists and social workers in the area studied, although elsewhere the system seems to work less well. Legally, the system may be unfair; these patients did not appear on the records as having been officially detained nor, presumably, were they told of the law which allows for such detention. On the other hand, they may have benefited in terms of the speed of response and the quality of service.

The police as diagnosticians of the mentally ill

The 1983 Act says a constable can detain a patient 'who appears to him to be suffering from mental disorder and to be in immediate need of care and control'. This means the police have to make decisions about mental disorder and be diagnosticians (not entirely, of course, for – once detained – the patient will be seen by those more formally qualified but, even so, an initial diagnosis is made by the police). It is, of course, true that the police have no formal training in these matters and, on the face of it, it would appear to make little sense for an unqualified layman to pronounce on medical matters. However, under Section 136, the police are required to make a low-level diagnosis. That is they have to decide whether the patient is in need of care and control which becomes as much a social and moral exercise as a psychiatric one.

Even so, it appears that the police are rather good at making this type of low-level diagnosis. In my own research, all patients detained by the police were, with one exception, compulsorily admitted to the mental hospital by the visiting consultant psychiatrist (Bean, 1980). The exception was a patient well known to the mental hospital who had a note on his hospital file stating that on no account should he be readmitted as his behaviour in the past had been too disruptive. The psychiatrist agreed that the patient currently suffered from mental disorder but he refused admission and the patient was diverted to the penal system and charged with threatening behaviour. The Butler Committee also noted that the police were efficient sources of referral and quoted a study by H. Rollin where, in the vast majority of cases, police action was shown to be fully justified. Another quoted study by Gibbens concluded that the police almost never act wrongly in bringing cases under Section 136; indeed Gibbens also points out that figures for previous admissions suggest that the police knew much of the patient's psychiatric history anyway (HMSO, 1975, paras 9.10–9.12).

Other studies show similar results. Kelleher & Copeland (1972) for example studied 92 admissions under Section 136 and compared these with 208 compulsory admissions by medical practitioners. They found that the police were as efficient at recognising persons in need of psychiatric care as were medical practitioners. The authors concluded that 'if certain criteria are valid indicators of correct use' such as the use of the emergency order, the use of Section 25 (the 28 day order under the 1959 Act), length of time in hospital etc, 'then the police do marginally better than other professionals'. Sims & Symonds (1975) also studied psychiatric referrals from the police, although not under Section 136, and found that the police tended to refer a high percentage of psychotic patients, of which 40% were diagnosed as suffering from schizophrenia. These studies go some way to confirming results found elsewhere which show the police are able to diagnose psychiatric patients as effectively as other professionals (see also Berry & Orwin, 1966; Mountney, Freyes & Freeman, 1969).

These studies have been listed in some detail if only to show that the police were reasonably efficient as diagnosticians of mental disorder. It is interesting to speculate why this should be so. It may be that their expertise stems from considerable experience in dealing with people who show bizarre and odd behaviour. Perhaps the police learn quickly to separate offenders into various categories. Dealing with the sad and the bad they learn also to distinguish the mad as well. Their skills are borne of experience and based on their close associations with the less benevolent in our society.

If the police are such competent and efficient sources of referral one would have thought that would go in their favour. This is apparently not the case, for the argument gets tied into other arguments, where professional rivalries exist and where ideological positions are asserted and fought over. On matters of professional rivalry, social workers for example are critical of the police because they say the police lack the professional training of social workers and are therefore unable to deal sensitively with the mentally ill. The police, in retaliation, merely assert that social workers do not have a monopoly of sensitivity in this matter. (The police also point out that social workers did not appear to be sufficiently sensitive to dispense with the more robust police approach when their erstwhile sensitivity fails to produce the desired results and the patients require physical control.) Social workers' criticisms of the police do not however extend to taking over the police role for, like it or not, no other occupational group could, or would be willing to take that over.

The Butler Commission put it this way: 'Where some action has to be taken to deal with a disordered individual in a public place it is better for the police to cope rather than a doctor or social worker whose authority may not be so readily recognised and who may not be quickly on the scene in an emergency' (HMSO, 1975, para. 9.7). The committee could have added that the police tend to patrol on a 24 hour basis and in areas of our cities where few others would be prepared to go. That alone makes them obvious candidates for operating Section 136. The police also have powers of arrest which are not conferred on others. The Butler Committee noted in this respect that there are certain common law powers of arrest which social workers or medical practitioners could use, but suggested these powers are obscure and should not be relied upon (HMSO, 1975).

Opposition to Section 136 also occurs within groups holding strong ideological positions which in turn tend to be bound up with a wider debate about the role of the police within society (or more specifically about the police and their relationships with cetain minority groups – mainly blacks). One can see how the argument unfolds. Historically, provisions of one sort or another for enabling the mentally disordered to be taken to a place of safety can be traced back to the Criminal Lunatics Act of 1800 and the 1885 Act (Walker & McCabe, 1973, vol. 2 Appendix A). The Poor Law was designed in part to solve a law and order problem of the nineteenth century. It is said that Section 136 is used to solve the law and order problem of the twentieth century. This time it is directed towards minority groups, notably blacks, instead of the maladjusted working class whites of earlier times. Whether so or not, one can see also how this debate gets tied into a second debate about the relationship between police and the blacks generally, and the fear and distrust blacks have of being detained by police, especially in police stations.

Yet, as far as can be seen from the official figures, whilst blacks tend to be overrepresented they are not unfairly so (or rather, not in a way that suggests the police are detaining blacks who are not mentally disordered). There are many reasons why blacks might be overrepresented. The main one, I suggest, is that deviance amongst mentally disordered blacks is more visible: it takes place in the streets. One could then postulate a labelling-type argument where the police detain and social workers and medical practitioners give credibility to the police decisions. Yet blacks are not the only group claiming to be overrepresented and, by implication, dealt with unfairly. Certain womens' organisations make similar claims. In 1982, however, out of the 1885 persons officially detained under Section 136, 1049 were men (or about 60%) and 836 (40%) were women. In an unreported study at one of the London mental hospitals in 1983 of 117 patients detained under Section 136, 60% were male and 40% female. Now of course these figures show women to be underrepresented, when 40% of those detained are women (women represent 51% of the population generally). Womens' organisations make comparisons, however, with the crime figures; these show that only about 25% of detained offenders are women. The crime figures helps, make the case they say, implying that the police are directing additional energy to the mentally disordered woman rather than to criminal women, or that they are evaluating womens' behaviour differently. Whether so or not, much more needs to be known before the argument becomes credible.

There are limits anyway as to the amount to be learned from these official figures not least because they deal mainly with the Metropolitan district of London. The proposed solutions are much more interesting. It is worthwhile to note however that much of the sting could have been drawn from criticisms of Section 136 had Parliament accepted the Percy Commission's recommendations some 30 years ago. (HMSO, 1957). The Commission thought it important that the patient be detained in a hospital rather than a police station; the commission said 'compel him to go to a hospital if he is unwilling' (HMSO, 1957, para. 4.12) although it is not entirely clear what would happen if the hospital then refused admission. Moreover the commission also recommended that the police should 'detain the patient only if his behaviour is such that he is liable to arrest under normal police powers' (HMSO, 1957) presumably by causing a breach of the peace or some such similar offence. Parliament did not accept these proposals, preferring to give the police wider powers allowing detention to take place in a police station and allowing the police to detain where no offence has been committed. Critics of Section 136, particularly those from minority groups, have always claimed that the discretion granted to the police permits discrimination to be practised under mental health legislation.

Most of the criticisms of Section 136 centre on two major areas: first, the responsibility for detaining the patient; second, the place where the patient should be detained. For the first, the more radical and extreme view is to argue (as some do) that Section 136 should be abolished. Those favouring this do not doubt that there are mentally disordered patients in public places and that they should be detained. They would prefer such patients to be taken directly to hospital by medical and ambulance staff without legal or police intervention. That would seem to provide no solution at all; if anything it would compound, aggravate and perhaps exacerbate the problem. It means, in effect, making medical and ambulance staff surrogate police officers. Would they accept this and would medical and allied staff also be prepared to patrol on a 24 hour basis? I think not. Would they also be prepared to undertake all that is involved in detaining difficult aggressive patients, even if they were granted powers of arrest similar to those given to the police? Again, I think not. Would they also be prepared to use the ambulance as an acceptable place of safety, and what would happen if, after all this, the hospital refused admission? As was said earlier, there are many good reasons why the police have to be seen as the one group likely to (and indeed able to) detain patients, or to be the point of first contact for these mentally disordered persons.

There is a more considered argument, less strident and more worthy of examination (although I think it too has serious defects): that is, the police should retain their existing powers to stop and detain patients but – as soon as possible thereafter – hand the patient over to others (such as medical and ambulance staff) who would then transfer and hold the patient in the place of safety. This should always be a hospital, never a police station. Contact between the police and patients would therefore be reduced, it is said. Supposedly, this would provide benefits for certain minority groups and help ease racial tension. The argument hinges on a wish to avoid contact with the police or minimise it as far as possible. I respect these views, yet, at the same time, this type of proposal is not without certain practical difficulties, some of which incidentally are given above. First, it is not clear if medical and ambulance men would wish to take on these extra duties. Second, there is an assumption which I find unable to accept that certain political and social problems can be reduced or eradicated if they become medicalised. It is an assumption based on the view that the police is the only occupational group which is prejudiced, or rather that it is more prejudiced than medical and allied staff. It also implies that medicalising a problem reduces conflict and tension. Medical and allied staff do not have unblemished records in matters of prejudice (although I suppose it could be argued they may be less prejudiced than the police, but, even this is not proved). Moreover, conflict or prejudice is not necessarily reduced under a medical canopy; often it reappears in more covert forms. When such conflict or prejudice exists it is no less easy to resolve, being sustained by structural features linked to professional attitudes and reinforced by institutional supports.

The second area for reform concerns the place of safety itself, that is the place where the patient should be so detained. The police have been advised by the Home Office *Consolidated Circular to the Police on Crime and Kindred Matters* (see HMSO, 1975, Appendix 7), that a person who is removed under this section should normally be taken direct to a hospital or, if this is not practicable, that the assistance of a social worker should be sought immediately. The duties of the social worker in this are, according to the Butler Report (HMSO, 1975, para. 9.1).

contacting the detained persons relatives and ascertaining whether there is a history of psychiatric treatment. Should admission to hospital prove necessary such information gathered by the social worker may indicate which hospital would be most suitable; but the social worker and to some extent the medical practitioner should always consider whether any course other than admission to hospital is appropriate. Knowing the range of resources which is available the social worker is in a position to assess all the circumstances and is responsible for making sure whether treatment in hospital is the only solution.

In spite of such a strong recommendation and perhaps because of practical difficulties things do not work quite like that. No one is sure how often the police use the police station as a place of safety, for they are not required to provide this information. It is suspected, however, that the advice given in the Home Office circular may not often be taken and a police station is used frequently. One can see why. The police may regard the patient as too aggressive or disturbed to keep their options open and charge the patient with an offence if he is not admitted to a hospital. The police station is more appropriate therefore under these circumstances. Moreover, the social worker is not always the first to be called – in my research it was the psychiatrist and the police medical officer who saw the patient first (Bean, 1980). The police have to gauge the likely social worker and medical response and they may well regard the police station as offering them the best and more predictable form of control.

There is no doubt however that detention in a police station under Section 136 causes great concern to many minority groups. Various solutions have been offered, one of which is for purpose-built institutions to be provided, staffed and controlled by local authorities. There is no objection to this in principle, assuming that local authorities were prepared to provide such facilities. Local authorities however may be less enthusiastic about taking on such a task. It would be expensive and would mean making their employees custodians. There would be no legal difficulty however for such powers already exist. Section 137(2) says that

Any other person authorised by or by virtue of this act to take into custody or to convey or detain any person shall, for the purpose of taking him into custody or conveying him have all the powers authorities protection or privileges which a constable has within the area for which he acts as constable.

And Section 137(1) says that when a person is so detained he shall be deemed to be in legal custody with all that means in terms of powers granted to those who have to retake those who escape etc. (Section 138). The objections may well therefore be on financial, social and moral grounds.

Yet there is an assumption contained in the proposal that the patient would be less vulnerable if detained in local authority accommodation. I am not sure this is so. Some patients may well feel less intimidated but would they all be provided with adequate standards of care, be given the appropriate protection from other such patients and be provided with medical and legal advice? Would local authorities provide less-than-adequate standards, bearing in mind current financial restraints? Would it greatly affect the nature of detention? Whatever the place or the custodian, detention is as real whether custodians be in uniform or not. I suggest however, a different approach. It may in the long run be more important to re-examine the service provisions, including the link between the police and the social and medical professions than be too concerned about the place of safety. Were services to be improved I suspect other improvements would follow.

Section 136: an overview

Section 136 provides powers of detention. It is a hybrid Section, not being a means of detaining patients in hospital for treatment but detaining them before a decision can be made. It places the police in a difficult position but they seem not to object. In fact the Association of Chief Police Officers, in evidence to the Butler Committee (HMSO, 1975, para. 9.7) was strongly opposed to its repeal. For that I think we must be relieved; there are no adequate substitutes or none that come to mind. We may accept this yet may still be critical about the length of time to be detained, the place of safety itself, the police's relationships with minority groups and above all the lack of a standardised procedure which does not involve the police making records of all patients they detain.

All societies require some mechanism or procedure to deal with mentally disordered persons found in public places and Section 136 is the method chosen in England and Wales. It relies on cultural expectations and a benign form of policing. It would work less well and probably not at all if that form of policing changed to a more aggressive, conflict-orientated, state-directed system. Mental health legislation would inevitably be seen then as a naked tool for the suppression of unacceptable views. The police in Britain operate relatively benignly and detain those who ought to be detained; this allows them to remain free from the more severe criticism. There is above all little or no evidence to suggest they railroad people into places of detention. Yet constant monitoring is required. Moreover, Section 136 has been a neglected area of interest where research might throw light on some puzzling features. Why, for instance, is the use of Section 136 largely restricted to London?

In 1973, for example, Wales recorded 10 patients detained under Section 136; the Merseyside Region, 1 (HMSO, 1975, para. 9.4). Why are there such wide variations? When used elsewhere, are there certain police areas which resemble the Metropolitan district in the manner in which they record patients, or are other practices used? Whatever the answer, there seems good reason to insist on more rigorous and standard procedures. A possible solution is to insist as some MPs did in the parliamentary debates on the 1983 Act that the police record patients on Section 136 at the point of detention and not (as sometimes appears at present) when the patient is admitted, having been seen by the social worker and registered medical practitioner.

Whilst it may be important to insist on a more rigorous set of procedures, matters of substance ought not to be so neglected. We know little of the professional negotiations that take place between police and the social workers or psychiatrists. At a conference organised by MIND in October 1984, one speaker showed how a police station serving two London boroughs reported 16 patients detained under Section 136 for the Borough of Brent but only 2 from Harrow over the same period. The critical variable was not, he suggested, the activities of the police but rather those of the social workers and medical officers. In Brent the police found professional assistance more forthcoming. In Harrow patients were detained and a Section 136 order was made only when the social workers and psychiatrists agreed to see the patients (which they did rarely). When they did not agree, the patients were not recorded under Section 136, but were dealt with in other ways (perhaps charged with a criminal offence or released). Elsewhere it seems practice differs again: in other London boroughs, a Section 136 order is made on the patient after he has been accepted in a hospital; the police, after detaining the patient in a police station, are advised to bring him to the local mental hospital where he is seen accordingly. If he is admitted, a Section 136 order is made; if not, the patient is otherwise dealt with.

It is difficult to generalise, but one theme begins to emerge; that is the variability of the service offered to the police by social and medical allied staff (Rassaby and Rogers, 1986). Unhappily too that service is often tinged with professional rivalries and distrust. The police see the medical and allied staff promoting unnecessary opposition and providing a less-than-efficient service when patients are detained. The police also complain of being dealt with in a churlish and patronising way by medical staff, having been encouraged to bring the patient to a local mental hospital at some cost in police time and manpower, and then being dismissed in a perfunctory and discourteous manner. They complain too of an anti-police ideology amongst some social workers and medical practitioners.

Of themselves, those professional rivalries are of little importance. They are endemic to the system although, to an outsider, they may seem petty and unseemly. Unfortunately they cannot do other than adversely affect the patients and reduce the quality of the service. Early contacts by the police with the mentally disordered and the quality of the service provided have repercussions which send ripples throughout other parts of the system, notably the prisons and the regional secure units (RSUs). For, as will be shown in Chapter 6, the prison system takes a large number of mentally disordered offenders and is unable to provide the necessary treatment for them. The police, finding that the services offered to them under Section 136 are less-than-adequate, may prefer the more simple approach: to charge the offender with a public order offence and let the courts decide. Inevitably, some of those patients will then find their way into the prison system. Better services from medical and social work staff may prevent this, to the advantage of all concerned.

We ought not to believe that Section 136 is likely to fade away although, ideally, I suppose primary health care systems could be developed which avoid police involvement. If anything, the trend is towards greater police activity. In London it is generally the large psychiatric hospitals, some of which are due for closure, to which mentally disordered people are removed for assessment. The question arises as to what alternative facility is best able to provide the necessary service. It is also clear from the programmes of community-based mental health services elsewhere that deinstitutional-isation results in increasing calls upon the police to provide a primary mental health service. This makes it all the more important that police act appropriately in dealing with mentally disordered people, that there is proper liaison between police and other services, particularly with the primary health care service, and that there are adequate facilities for providing necessary assessment and care.

Often deinstitutionalisation means the absence of primary health care. This is so in Britain and perhaps elsewhere. The police are forced thereby into the front line, as it were. Yet, as matters stand, there are few facilities for the police to develop skills with the mentally disordered. In fact the system often works in the opposite direction. Police rarely receive feedback from the hospital about their referrals or, indeed, whether the patient was admitted or not. It is not uncommon for the police to be called to take a person to hospital when they have already taken him there days, or even hours, before. Lack of coordination between the police and health services, including GPs is a major problem in itself but it makes matters more difficult for the police if they are to evaluate their methods. It is too simple to say the police ought to be better trained, when they find that training produces little in the form of direct returns.

At the wider policy level, the question is how to equip primary health care systems with the means to identify the mentally disordered and to reduce as far as possible pressures on the police to intervene where others have failed. In part I suppose there could be more efficient community-based assessment facilities but, given the current climate of public service provisions, one should not I think rely on these being developed. One could hope too that sections of the primary health care services, the GPs for example, may make a greater contribution but doubts remain there too. The fear is that the police will be increasingly involved against a backdrop of the closure of mental hospitals and the professional rivalries that take place throughout the system.

Section II

Control of patients in the hospital and community

CHAPTER 5

Guardianship and control in the community

Historically the power to make a guardianship order was derived from the ancient concept of *parens patriae* where the guardian looked after and cared for those who could not care for themselves. Later guardianship, like so much else in modern health legislation, became bound up with the Poor Law, at least for the less well off. It was developed by the 1913 Mental Deficiency Act and later by the 1959 Mental Health Act where it was refined and extended, though hardly ever used. Under the 1983 Act, the major provisions of which can be found in Sections 7–10, guardianship has been retained although, under this Act, there are restricted powers of the guardian. These restrictions were introduced in order to encourage greater use: this is not a paradox, for it was thought that the guardian's earlier powers were excessive and represented too much of an imposition on the patient. However, as will be shown later, this in my view is an oversimplification; in spite of changes, guardianship is no more popular than hitherto.

One can see how guardianship and the Poor Law were linked. Guardianship means the supervision by one person, the appointed guardian, over the patient. The Poor Law guardians were responsible for those unable to care for themselves and, as mentally disordered people often required supervised care, the duties of the guardian were assumed. Moreover those requiring care were often mentally defective children, hence guardianship was seen to be more a matter for the Mental Deficiency Act (Sections 3, 5 and 6 were the major sections) than the 1890 Lunacy Act. Persons subject to guardianship could be detained in an asylum as well as being supervised in the community. If in an asylum, then, the guardian had to approve and, once detained, the patient had to be visited at least once a year by a medical practitioner with experience in mental deficiency, and at least twice a year by officers of the local health authority or some other approved person. Such was the influence of legalism and the demands that detained patients should receive legal protection, although how effective this was in practice is not known. The basic concept remained; that is, the guardian had a legal and moral duty to care for those unable to care for themselves.

It has been said in Chapter 2 that modern legislation in mental health is dependent on earlier legislation and this is particularly true of guardianship. It is so in detail and in conception. In the first, the functions and powers of those operating that legislation have remained largely unchanged. New legislation has tended to be translated into older moral directives into up-to-date structures using modern idioms and language. So, instead of the Poor Law guardians, we have the local authority whilst the Poor Law relieving officer has been replaced by the Approved Social Worker. Moreover, under the 1913 Act, approved practitioners made medical recommendations; this is also the case under the 1983 Act. The basic mixture of care and control has been retained as before. There may be new justifications, there may even be new forms of language but these serve only to mask the essential sameness. Guardianship remains what it always was; a device to care for patients needing care, and to control patients needing control whether they be offenders or non-offenders alike. Those who framed the Poor Law recognised the importance of those two features, so too apparently did those framing the 1983 Act although the control element has tended to be played down. If anything, guardianship under the 1983 Act has moved closer to its Poor Law predecessors – and, in saying this, I am not implying any criticism, merely describing trends.

Guardianship under the 1959 Act

In its conception guardianship was extended under the 1959 Act and modified 24 years later. Those modifications have been seen by some as restricting the vision of guardianship while, for others, as necessary reforms to encourage greater use. Guardianship has always retained its supporters, offering as it does the opportunity to care for the patient without recourse to direct hospitalisation. The Percy Commission preceding the 1959 Act recognised this and it was their vision of guardianship that has dominated. The detail they provided has been criticised as being too restrictive but the mechanics have been loyaly retained. (HMSO, 1957).

The Percy Commission wanted *inter alia* to promote legislation on the basis of two major premises. First, that there should be a unified set of legal provisions for all mentally disordered. Hitherto guardianship had been largely for mentally defective patients, but the commission saw this as producing rigid legal and administrative barriers which prevented patients receiving appropriate care. Treatment, said the commission, should be according to patients needs (para. 188) and diagnosis and classification should indicate suitable forms of care based on current demands. Unhappily, said the commission, the term 'defective' had become pejorative and permanent, it should therefore be replaced by new terminology adjusted and evaluated on the basis of the current illness. 'Subnormality', or even 'severe subnormality' were seen to be better, themselves forms of mental disorders (and of course replaced under the 1983 Act with mental and severe mental impairment). Even so, the commission did not want to restrict guardianship to patients in those diagnostic categories but for it to be applied to the mentally disordered generally. If those mentally disordered were also offenders, then so be it; guardianship was to be for all, offenders and non-offenders alike.

One can see the logic of this and it fitted well into the commission's view of things. This was to be only the first step. The second was equally important, for the commission linked guardianship to community care. The commission argued that community care should be given if, and only if the patient could be pursuaded to cooperate with officers of the local health authority and accept their help, advice, and the arrangements made for employment occupation and training (para. 399). (Of course the commission's definitions of community care is a restricted one, by modern standards, equating as it does community care with local authority provision and with employment occupation and training, but never mind.) If there was no cooperation then compulsory powers may justifiably be used to place the patient under guardianship (para. 399). Or, in other words, guardianship was to be used as a form of compulsion to guarantee community care for those who would choose otherwise.

The commission expected that those subject to guardianship would be patients with mild forms of mental disorder not needing to be in hospital. They might also include some elderly people requiring a form of residential care in local authority homes not covered by Section 47 of the National Assistance Act 1948.[1] Guardianship was for patients who could be maintained in the community where the guardian would control the place of residence, employment, and use of earnings to ensure appropriate training and care. More than that, those on guardianship might require short periods in hospital, said the commission, thereby drawing heavily on the old Poor Law legislation. If so, then those patients could be transferred to hospital if necessary (paras 466–8); a proposal incidentally accepted by Parliament, introduced into the 1959 Act but, in practice, rarely used. Sometimes the opposite may be required, that is, patients in hospital might benefit from guardianship. The commission proposed that such patients could be transferred to guardianship not more than 6 months after leaving hospital, if proper after care could not be guaranteed by other means. The commission wanted to provide an integrated system of care with guardianship as a mid-point between various extremes. 'Viewing the mental health services as a whole hospital treatment should now be regarded as a stage which is commonly preceded and followed by some form of community care or out patient treatment' (para. 668). As to the powers of the guardian, the commission recommended they should be equivalent to the powers of a parent over a child – which meant a 14 year old child according to the 1959 Act (Section 34(1)).

These proposals were introduced by the commission in a spirit of optimism. The commission expected that they would provide an additional measure to be used by the courts and psychiatrists alike which was integrated into the general provisions of compulsory powers. Like so much else in the commission's report, its proposals were accepted by Parliament in like manner. Briefly the 1959 Act providing the following: guardianship was defined in Section 33 as being for a patient suffering from mental disorder, that is of any age for mental illness or severe subnormality but under the age of 21 for psychopathic disorder and subnormality. This was necessary in order to bring guardianship into line with the treatment order (Section 26) since treatment could also be provided on the guardianship order. An order for guardianship was to be made on the grounds that it was necessary in the interests of the patient or for the protection of other persons that the patient should be so received (Section 33(2)(6)). The named guardian had to be either a local health authority or any other person but, if the latter, then the order had no effect unless it was accepted by the local health authority (Section 33(3)). Section 34(1) conferred on the guardian the appropriate powers, that was that the guardian should (to the exclusion of any other person) have powers as would be exercisable in relation to the patient if he were the father of the patient and the patient was under the age of 14 years. Section 34(5) provided the patient with the right to apply to a Mental Health Review Tribunal within 6 months of being on guardianship, thereby bringing guardianship further into line with the existing treatment order. Section 43(1) stated the length of time under guardianship; that was 1

Year	Numbers on guardianship	New cases	Numbers of local authorities not returning figures to the DHSS
1981	153	56	10
1982	164	47	9
1983	163	47	10

Source: DHSS, personal communication.

year in the first instance, but renewable in the same manner as with Section 26 the treatment order. Section 44(1) provided special provisions as to psychopathic patients and subnormal patients, that is guardianship should cease to have effect for them once they reached the age of 25 years.

In spite of the commission's and Parliament's enthusiasm, guardianship did not become that fulcrom in the compulsory care system. In fact it was used rather infrequently as shown in the above table.

Nor did it appear to be used for the offender patients either where, under Section 60 of the 1959 Act, a court could (subject to certain conditions being satisfied) order an offender to be placed under guardianship. That order lasted also for 12 months. The Butler Committee on the Mentally Abnormal Offender (HMSO, 1975) saw guardianship as having 'evident value'. The committee recognised that guardianship was to some extent competing with probation orders as a sentencing option and particularly those probation orders which had a condition of psychiatric treatment attached. The committee recognised too that probation orders had the advantage of allowing the probation officer to bring the offender back to court. Moreover the probation service had the advantage of close cooperation with the Courts where probation officers could, and often did, offer opinions as to the suitability of the offender for this or that type of sentence. Even so the Butler committee clearly approved of the principle of guardianship: 'It is our view that guardianship offers a useful form of control of some mentally disordered offenders who do not require hospital treatment; and particularly suited to the needs of subnormal offenders' (HMSO, 1975, para. 15.8). It cited case histories where, under the supervision of the guardian patients improved. Some were helped to find suitable employment, others given training; for others the provision of hostel accommodation was said to have had a stabilising effect. Some patients also were said to be more successful in managing their financial affairs as a result of being on a guardianship order, and there was, said the committee, evidence to suggest success in reducing re-admission (para. 15.3). Given these apparent advantages, the committee said it was surprised to see how little use was made of guardianship for offender patients. In

1971, 11 offenders were placed on a guardianship order in England and Wales, 4 in 1972, 8 in 1973 and 7 in 1974 (para. 15.4). (In fact these figures had already shown a steady decrease since 1961, the first full year guardianship operated when 21 offenders were placed on such orders.) However, perhaps the enthusiasm expressed by the Butler Committee was carried over to the courts and others, for the numbers increased in 1981 to 22 and there were a further 22 and 17 placed on guardianship in 1982 and 1983 respectively.

It is all the more surprising therefore that the Butler Committee made no firm recommendations for change. 'We do not think there is a need for statutory alternatives with regard to the present system of guardianship orders but we would encourage the close liaison between the Courts and social services departments of local authorities' (para. 15.8). Was this perhaps a lost opportunity? For, on the face of it, guardianship does appear to have something to offer even if in a negative sense – that is, to keep the patient out of hospital. A case example from my own research illustrates the point – this example being from a series of non-offender patients.

A woman aged 35 had two small children under 5 years and was a single parent. She had been discharged two months earlier from a mental hospital with instructions to maintain herself on medication in order to stabilise her schizophrenic condition. She had stopped taking the medication, her earlier symptoms had returned and she and her children were in some distress. The consultant psychiatrist recommended a guardianship order but the local authority social worker refused to agree on the basis that her social service department did not accept guardianship as a matter of policy. The patient was compulsorily readmitted and the children taken into care.

Bean (1980).

It is instructive to note in this example that the local authority in question (Nottinghamshire) has not had one guardianship order since guardianship had been introduced by the 1959 Act. Had such an order been made in the case cited above it is possible that the children would not have been taken into care, and compulsory hospitalisation would have been avoided. Surely worthwhile objectives in themselves on humanistic grounds if not psychiatric ones?

Guardianship under the 1983 Act

In the parliamentary debate on the 1983 Act member after member spoke of guardianship with enthusiasm – perhaps because it was associated with community care, another prescriptive term, and perhaps because it offered opportunities for a less expensive alternative to compulsory hospitalisation. Parliament's solution was to reduce the powers of the guardian, believing that powers equivalent to that over a 14 year old child were excessive. Also the time, energy and extent of contact required by local authorities was doubtless seen by some as unrealistic if the guardian was to exercise his powers fully, and yet be open to criticism if not. At the simple administrative level, it was perhaps unrealistic to expect local authorities to be prepared to take on a task which could be time consuming and expensive. It seemed certain to some MPs that local authorities might find a guardianship order more attractive if it were on the lines of a supervision or probation order – that is, involving less detailed supervision.

The result, under the 1983 Act, has been a modified order whilst retaining those earlier features of guardianship defined in previous legislation. The guardian under Section 8 of the 1983 Act has three specific powers. The first is to require the patient to live at the place specified by the guardian (Section 8(1)(a)). This, according to the DHSS, is to discourage the patient from sleeping rough or living with people who may exploit or mistreat him, or to ensure he resides in a particular hostel or other facility (DHSS, 1983 para. 46). The second power enables the guardian to require the patient to attend specified places at specified times 'for medical treatment, occupation, education or training but there is no power to make him accept treatment' (Section 8(1)(b)). (There are however powers to transfer a patient to hospital from guardianship – see Regulation 8(3).) Finally there are powers which enable the guardian to gain access to the patient, to be given at the place where the patient is living, to any doctor, Approved Social Worker or other person specified by the guardian (Section 8(1)(c)). This power could be used for example to ensure that the patient did not neglect himself (DHSS, 1983 para. 46).

The Act made other changes, some of which are important others less so. For example, under the 1983 Act, guardianship cannot now be used for anyone under the age of 16 years (Section 7(1)); the length of the order is now 6 months (Section 20(2)(a)) renewable for 6 months – rather than for 1 year, as before (Section 20(8)). These changes also add limitations to the guardian's powers and move the concept of guardianship further towards legalism. In addition, should the patient fail to cooperate or should he leave his residence without the guardian's permission, he can be taken into custody and brought back. After 28 days, the power to re-take the patient expired. This applies to all patients within the four principle categories of mental disorder – a change from the previous Act where patients suffering from psychopathic disorder or subnormality could be taken into custody for up to 6 months. There are no other sanctions should the patient fail to cooperate with the guardian, the existing ones are thought sufficient to allow the guardian to influence the patient and provide the necessary assistance. The DHSS called these the 'essential powers' approach, that is powers which restrict the liberty of the individual 'only to the extent necessary to ensure that various forms of medical treatment, social support, training or occupation are undertaken' (DHSS, 1978, para. 4.17). The 'essential powers' approach can be contrasted with other options available: first, the 'community care order' which would provide powers similar to that were the patient to be in hospital: second, the 'revised form of guardianship' which would merely tighten up existing definitions such as providing second opinions for treatments etc. The 'essential powers' approach was the one selected by Parliament. It provides a shift away from the view contained in the 1959 Act. That was defined as the more full-blooded version but thought in the 1980s to be too paternalistic and too restrictive and out of touch with the times.

How successful have these changes been? In terms of the number of patients placed on guardianship order in the first 12 months of operation of the 1983 Act, there has been a slight increase in its use, but no dramatic change. In the 6 months beginning 1 April 1983 there were 156 cases of guardianship in England and Wales, of which 26 were new cases. These figures may not give the full picture as 35 local authorities failed to complete returns. In the next 6 months there were 177 cases, of which 34 were new ones with 14 local authorities not completing returns. For the offender patients under Section 37, in those first 6 months there were 20 offenders under guardianship (4 of whom were new ones). In the next 6 months, there were 18 offenders on guardianship and another 4 were new. So, a slight increase has been recorded, but hardly substantial and almost irrelevant when taken as a percentage of inpatient admissions, compulsory or otherwise.

The reason for the continued lack of interest is, according to some local authorities that the new legislation has created additional obstacles, and they cite ambiguities in the drafting relating to the duties of the guardian. By implication, they say minor changes in the drafting will make all the difference. I think this is not the whole story. Minor changes will not deal with the main problem, for I am sure that is financial. That is, guardianship is a costly exercise and has to compete with other service provisions at a time of central government cutbacks. Guardianship costs the local authorities money even though it may save money for the NHS. Already some local authorities have expressed concern that guardianship might involve them in demands to provide sophisticated and costly alternative facilities in terms of staff and buildings. They have also stated publicly that existing manpower resources make it unlikely that social workers would be able to take on further specialist training that would be essential. These seem to be the main reasons for their lack of interest and minor amendments will not, I suspect, change that. Of course the fewer guardianship orders dealt with, the less experience the social workers will gain, and the less inclination to provide them in the future. It is a self-fulfilling exercise.

Guardianship and the ideology of entitlement

Assume for the moment that guardianship is prescriptive, and accept too the arguments given above, i.e. that local authorities fail to use guardianship because they are reluctant to spend money on the provision of those services. This then raises a more fundamental question defined in Gostin's terms as the 'ideology of entitlement' (Gostin, 1983). Gostin asserts that access to health or social services should not be based on discretion, charitable or professional claims but rather upon enforceable rights. Parliament is not obliged to pass legislation to provide health and social services but, if it does, it cannot arbitrarily deprive or exclude certain individuals or client groups. Translate this into terms of guardianship and we have the position where Parliament has provided facilities for patients, defined as good in themselves and therefore likely to be of benefit to those patients. For some reason or other those facilities are not being used or indeed provided; if they are, they are used infrequently or not at all. Larry Gostin's point is that such failures as there are should be remedied by law.

Could they be? Certainly the Secretary of State for Health and Social Services under the 1977 National Health Service Act (Sections 1–5) has overall responsibility for the promotion of a comprehensive health and social service to secure improvement in the physical and mental health of people in England and Wales and in the prevention, diagnosis and treatment of illness including mental disorder. He also has a duty to provide, to the extent he considers necessary, and to meet all reasonable requirements of hospital and other accommodation, services and facilities for the prevention, diagnosis and aftercare of persons who have been suffering from such illnesses. He does this by delegating powers and functions to Regional, District, or Special Health Authorities. Under Section 124(1) of the 1983 Act

where the Secretary of State is of the opinion on complaint or otherwise that a local social services authority have failed to carry out functions conferred or imposed on the authority by or under this Act or have in carrying out those functions failed to comply with any regulations relating to those functions, he may after such enquiry as he thinks fit make an order declaring the authority to be in default.

There are clearly provisions for the Secretary of State to order an inquiry and deem a local authority to be in default if those delegated powers are not carried out according to the appropriate requirements. On this basis, that particular local authority which has never accepted a guardianship order (from 1960 to 1983 or in the 12 months following the 1983 Act) is clearly in default. Gostin is thereafter correct: if there is unreasonable denial of a service (and, in this case, there would I suppose be evidence to support that), and the patient loses his rights, then the remedy is provided by law.

Lawyers tend to see matters in those terms. That is, the law is seen as providing rules which, in this case, produce rights for citizens and duties for local authorities. Rights that are violated are therefore, in lawyers' terms, open to remedy. Lawyers usually add to this a general principle which underpins those rights. In this instance, Gostin invokes the rules of equity and fairness which he says are deeply entrenched in common law. Equity and fairness in this case presumably mean that all patients have an equal opportunity to use that service. Services provided by local authority *A*, ought to be similarly provided by local authority *B*. Equity and fairness means comparability and commensurability.

Of course, at this basic level, Gostin is entirely correct. He wants to assert that the objective of the ideology of entitlement is to establish the right to a service which can be enforced at the behest of a client group. If Parliament provides such a service and local authorities fail to implement those provisions then the client group is, or should be, entitled to demand it. It matters not that this client group (the mentally disordered) is unable to demand it for itself, others can legitimately act on its behalf. The principle of equity and fairness states that the client group in whose area provisions were not forthcoming could claim that the local authority was in default.

Yet matters unfortunately are rarely as simple as that. For on what practical basis should the principle of equity and fairness operate? Should it be confined to the provision of basic services or perhaps extend to more rarefied and sophisticated ones? If the former, then the rules defining that service must be a good deal less open-ended than hitherto. They must distinguish between a duty and a recommendation. When the Percy Commission said it should be the duty of the local authorities to provide aftercare for all who need it, were they seriously expecting it should be a duty or were they making recommendations or scoring political points? More likely the last for, unless they defined clearly the nature of those services, the tendency is to see the statement as being of a high order of generality. It becomes interpreted as a statement of intent and perhaps a pious one at that.

Moreover, to say that a local authority has a duty to provide a service says nothing about the quality of that service. It may be that, as long as the bare bones or the rudiments are provided, the local authority can claim legitimately that it has performed its statutory duty. Guardianship, under these circumstances, may be available to all who need it but if, say, occupational training is limited, or if the guardian visits monthly rather than weekly or if residential requirements remain unenforced, or if medical attention is not forthcoming, there can hardly be a service in the accepted sense of that term. Yet as long as a service of some sort exists the local authority can claim to be fulfilling its duty. It can do other things too. It could provide a service in an area of a county where the population is low, where public services are poor and where it puts as many obstacles as possible in the path of those seeking the service. It can do all this and still claim it has provided a service.

Nor does that statement by the Percy Commission on aftercare, to use this example, say anything about the professional judgments required to determine whether this or that person qualifies for such a service. Professionals act as gatekeepers, letting some applicants through the gate, and refusing others. Sometimes those professionals act on the orders of their employers (as with, say, the attendance allowance paid to those unable to care for themselves – later, when more money became available, the professionals granted more allowances but patients earlier refused were no less in need). Sometimes professionals exclude applicants on the basis of their own professional judgments or provide a service defined in their terms which does not match the expectations of the recipients of that service. Numerous examples can be taken from medicine but an equally common one is in education where the quality of schools is determined as much by the professional's interpretation of their task as anything else. In social work, too, professional ideologies determine who are to be worthy recipients of a service and who not.

The principle of equity and fairness may even hinder matters. Equity may work very well for those having little, but not so well for those having rather more. If local authority *A* provides a guardianship service and local authority *B* does not, then (on the principle of equity and fairness) *B* should be compensated in some way. So far so good. If, however, local authority *A* provides a rather special type of guardianship service providing rather more than the basic requirements (say, it provides special facilities for sheltered employment) and local authority *B* provides the basic service, the principle of equity may well require local authority *A* to scale down its operations. Equity can be two-edged working to the benefit of those with little but to the detriment of those with the most. In saying this, no account needs to be taken of the efficiency of the service, defined as being appropriate to the patient; this too is a factor which adds to difficulties in legislating in this area. To speak of a 'right to a service' is to use the term 'right' in an entirely different way than say in the criminal law where rights are more specific, being less dependent on professional judgments and operate largely independent of needs.

Of course Gostin was not unaware of this. What he is trying to do is make local authorities provide services decreed by Parliament. So, if Parliament says guardianship is to be a means by which mentally disordered patients are to be cared for in the community and facilities for their care do not exist, then something is amiss. He sees the American system as more worthwhile where such rights are provided in State and Federal constitutions and he wishes to push Britain towards that system. Even if that were possible, and without a written constitution it seems hardly likely, many of the pitfalls mentioned above will still apply, i.e. those relating to professional judgments etc. There are limits to what legislation can achieve, a point which lawyers sometimes find it difficult to accept, but it remains true nonetheless. In acknowledging this I am not saying I disagree with the sentiment behind Gostin's proposal, merely that I remain less optimistic that results can be achieved by this approach. I hope I am not being too deeply cynical when I say I suspect there are some occasions when Parliament makes provisions and hopes they are never implemented. This may not be true of guardianship but may well be true of some others.

Perhaps after all, something can be salvaged from Gostin's ideology of entitlement. If so, I think there is a lesson to be taken from the welfare rights movement. The right to certain benefits have never been a 'right' in the usual sense of that term, but a privilege granted by Government. 'Welfare privileges' in this sense would have been a more accurate term. But welfare rights activists have constantly used the term 'rights' so much so that it has become almost as if those rights existed. Corresponding duties or claims made on these duties have been strengthened accordingly. The political lesson is a simple one: if claims to certain 'rights' are made sufficiently often they eventually appear as 'rights', and those rights are then said to exist. This seems to be the political message. In suggesting this we should not expect the courts to help for, on past performance (and to use Hoggett's phrase), English law cuts a pretty poor figure in this area. She says that having accepted the ideology of entitlement, the courts have largely abandoned its enforcement and left it to the politicians. They as we know, have found it hard to persuade themselves of the public good in developing services, whether it be for the mentally disordered or for others (Hoggett, 1984, p. 306)

Guardianship as a moral enterprise

Up to this point guardianship has been accepted as prescriptive, offering opportunities for the mentally disordered to be cared for in the community. It has also been seen as being under-used and, by implication, also seen as a more acceptable provision in the mental health field than hospitalisation. However, I think a note of caution should be added, as well as some criticism of the manner in which guardianship is devised and put into operation.

On the one hand, guardianship is entirely acceptable as an alternative to compulsory detention, though under the 1983 Act it is not seen as such. That is, it is not intended to be a community care order providing parallels with compulsory powers in a hospital – at least according to the official designation. It is an order aimed at ensuring care and protection for patients (DHSS, 1983, para. 45). Guardianship is nonetheless a control order limiting freedoms, even if for the most honourable of intentions. Insights obtained from criminology are instructive on this point. A new sentence introduced into the penal system finds its place on the tariff. This sentence attracts a group of offenders who would have been sentenced to a more severe sentence as well as a group who would have been sentenced to one less severe. So too may it be with guardianship. Some patients may be placed on guardianship who would otherwise have been detained compulsorily in mental hospitals but so too may some who are currently voluntary outpatients.

If certain measures are introduced or changed, i.e. local authorities are given financial assistance to help with guardianship orders, one could anticipate an increase in such orders. Indeed it would be strange if it were otherwise, for an order granting control in the community without the expense of hospitalisation could be extremely attractive (provided the local authorities were encouraged to underwrite the expense) The tendency to control the mentally disordered who present us with social and moral dilemmas, particularly if that encouragement is backed by financially attractive measures, would be hard for local authorities to resist. The more so as state mental hospitals are being cut back and more patients returned to the community. One could see a position where guardianship became extremely attractive, acting as an auxilary institution to the mental hospital. It could become another form of control and be capable of the widest interpretation.

As matters stand at the moment, guardianship *par excellence* contains that unwieldy mixture of the social, medical and moral. An application for guardianship must be founded on two medical recommendations, the procedure being similar to an application for admission for treatment. There are provisions for transfering a patient on guardianship to a hospital and from a hospital to guardianship – this in spite of the official disclaimers that guardianship is not an extension of the compulsory hospital system. Regulation 1 requires the guardian, if not a local social services authority, to appoint a doctor to act as a nominated medical attendant who will care for the patient's health. This doctor has the power to reclassify the patient and is responsible for examining the patient when the authority for his guardianship is due to expire and for making a report that the guardianship be renewed if appropriate. This responsible medical officer has the power of discharge in all cases, as do the local social services authority and the patient's nearest relative.

Essentially, the problems of guardianship are problems created by this unwieldy mixture of the social, medical and moral. The grounds for guardianship are that, amongst other things, 'it is in the interests of the welfare of the patient or for the protection of other persons' – a shift from the 1959 Act which said (author's stress) 'it is necessary in the *interests* of the patient or for the protection of other persons' (Section 33(2)(b)), created by the need to tighten up the drafting. How the term 'welfare' is thought to be superior to 'in the interests of' is difficult to understand. Even so, the rules relating to the renewal of guardianship require that the responsible medical officer says that it is necessary in the interests of the welfare of the patient, or for the protection of other persons, that the patient should remain under guardianship (Section 20(7)(b)). There could be no better illustration of a responsible medical officer acting as judge, jailer and moral protector all at the same time.

One may still ask what has 'the welfare of the patient' or 'the protection of other persons' to do with medicine anyway. That an application for guardianship is founded on two medical recommendations stating that a patient is suffering from one of the four types of mental disorder *and* it is necessary in the interests of his welfare to be received into guardianship is bad enough but something we shall have to live with as it differs hardly at all from the requirements relating to compulsory detention generally. Yet it still becomes a social and moral question. We may be able to accept with approval a statement on the patient's psychiatric condition, we may also be able to accept a view which says on the balance of probabilities patients with this or that condition tend to behave in this or that way. We ought not, however, to accept the idea that medical men should be encouraged to make pronouncements on matters which they (nor anybody else) can claim expertise. To do so is to continue the myth that the decision to curtail freedoms is based on the patient's mental condition and not on his behaviour, or that reliable diagnosis of that condition increases the predictive qualities of the diagnostician in terms of that behaviour. To repeat the point made in Chapter 3, we detain or control patients not for their psychiatric condition but for what they do and are likely to do. That must forever be a social and moral question.

The combination of medical, social and moral factors make guardianship a potential source of abuse. The Special Interest Group on Mental Health Issues of the British Association of Social Workers (BASW) illustrate that. The group listed a number of 'areas of concern'. These included a proposal that guardianship powers should be invoked to protect and control the elderly, mentally infirm both in hospital and in the community, limiting sanctions granted to the guardian to exercise powers, extending the amount of persuasion which could be used to direct clients to live in a particular place if they do not wish to cooperate, and examining the potential conflict between acting in the clients best interests and the demands of the role of guardian and advocate (*Social Work Today*, 15 July 1985). Some of these 'areas of concern' illustrate an interest in the patient's rights and freedoms (the latter, for example), yet others would increase the powers of the social work guardian. At best, they illustrate a depth of confusion, but also show how guardianship can readily be shifted to extend control. To be fair to the government, it recognised this, for in rejecting proposals for 'Community Care Orders' which would run parallel to compulsory hospital powers it saw 'the extent of control which community care orders would entail as being so wide that this option might well suffer the same disadvantages as guardianship has in the past' (DHSS, 1978, para. 4.16). Hence its choice of the 'essential powers' approach limited to 'restricting the liberty of the individual only to the extent necessary to ensure the various forms of medical treatment, social support, training, or occupations are undertaken' (DHSS, 1978, para. 4.17). It is a pity therefore that the government was not more careful in the legislation it promoted; that is, it should have produced tighter legal definitions further restricting the use and the power of the guardian.

As matters stand at present, guardianship can still produce detailed measures of control. If a patient is directed to reside in a specified place, the patient must also abide by the regulations and rules of that institution (which may be no less restrictive than a mental hospital and, perhaps, more so). The guardian has powers to require the patient to attend places and at times so specified for the purpose of medical treatment and, whilst the guardian cannot consent to treatment on the patient's behalf, opportunities for persuasion obviously exist. It is the guardian's duty to protect those who are exploited and cannot protect themselves.

There is nothing wrong with this, in principle, and much to applaud in provisions which allow people to live in the community rather than a hospital. I welcome too, official provisions which give assistance to those unable to protect themselves and remain likely to be exploited. One could say then that, on the face of it, guardianship is a humanistic device able to offer a great deal to a certain type of mental patient. Unfortunately, that which begins as a humanistic exercise can all too often develop into an extensive control system or (in the case of guardianship) as an auxiliary mental hospital. In the current climate, which involves a run down of mental hospitals and an enthusiasm for community care one can see guardianship assuming a more prominent position, attracting more funds, and being increasingly justified as an alternative to mental hospitals. It is not happening at the moment, as the number of guardianship orders shows, but it could do in the future given the obvious financial advantages. Such a demand would also fit the accepted view that solutions to social problems can be found in the provision of services and, should those services involve a compulsory element, then so be it. I wish to challenge that assumption and insist that guardianship be used rarely, even perhaps for short periods not exceeding 1 month, and that the law should be more specific about its use, and equally specific about the powers of the guardian. The alternative to one control system ought not to be to provide another, however well-intentioned that may be.

CHAPTER 6

The mentally disordered offender and professional dominance

Mental health legislation sits astride two control systems, the psychiatric and the penal, yet the two systems have different methods and aims. One is concerned with treating mentally disordered according to the medical paradigm, the other with inflicting suffering according to the principles of retribution or deferrence – depending on one's philosophical view of punishment (see Bean, 1981). One claims a scientific approach, the other is avowedly moral. One emphasises clinical judgments borne out of the expertise of the physician, the other the requirements of procedural rules and the evaluation of evidence within the dictates of judicial authority. The control systems touch at the points where the mentally disordered commit crimes or where criminals become mentally disordered, requiring each system to accommodate the other.

It was once fashionable to claim that all criminals were mentally disordered, neurotic perhaps rather than psychotic, and that treatment rather than punishment should dominate. Few seriously entertain such views nowadays although strands of that argument appear after the commission of certain heinous and bizarre crimes. Then, it is suggested, the criminal must be mentally deranged in some way. Mental disorder thus becomes associated with incredulity and mindless crime. Other than that, the general view is that most criminals are free from mental disorder and most mentally disordered are free from criminality. Whereas it was once fashionable to assert the 'crime of punishment' nowadays criminologists are more likely to talk of the 'crime of treatment' – the former on the basis that suffering should be substituted by treatment, the latter that treatment offers indeterminacy in sentencing and loss of procedural safeguards.

In Chapter II I will argue that law and psychiatry come from different epistemological traditions and the control systems reflect this. Indeed commentators such as Foucult (1978) insist that the tensions between those traditions produce rivalry and competition for power. He notes the extensive influence of psychiatry, whether it be through the treatment of prisoners in the penal system, the claims by psychiatry to provide categories of disorder for corresponding legal categories (kleptomania for theft, pyromania for arson, etc.), or the manner in which psychiatric explanations of behaviour have permeated the legal system. He uses the example of an offender appearing at court who bemused and confused everyone by refusing to give an explanation for his offences according to his background or personal relationships. Were psychiatry to dominate, Foucault fears there would be a loss of essential freedoms produced by the rule of law over centuries; (such as the right to plead, to cross-examine witnesses, to appeal against conviction or sentence, etc). In its place would be clinical judgments, and executive powers, the latter allowing treatment officials to pronounce on treatments dictated by the patient's condition rather than the offence. There would also be a different moral tradition where the offender (or patient) occupies the centre stage to the detriment of the victim and to social order generally.

It is not necessary to defend or attack Foucult's position but rather to see it as a hyperbole which provides the boundaries to the current debate. Foucault however is correct in this respect: the current professional rivalry between lawyers and psychiatrists cannot be explained at the level of a disagreement centring on the welfare of the patient. The intensity of that rivalry suggests something deeper and more extreme. Moreover to see psycholegal disagreements as friendly professional rivalries ignores too a debate which has dominated criminology for over a decade. That debate has illustrated the divisions between justice and treatment. Supporters of justice, or the justice model as it is often called, pull out and unmask the nature of treatment emphasising the loss of essential freedoms and the insecurities promoted by the exercise of executive powers. On the one hand the justice model, which draws upon the links between the crime and the sentence does not (and cannot) try to provide explanations of the offenders behaviour. Rather it emphasises the importance of the determinate sentence set in advance according to the legal statutes. It emphasises too the importance of an independant judiciary, the right of appeal and adherence to procedural rules. In contrast the treatment model emphasises the personal life of the offender, the nature of his social and psychological condition, and the benefit to be gained through treatment. It is against this background that the mentally abnormal offender must find his place where tensions of various kinds exist and uncertainty about the aims of the legislation is commonplace. Or as Hoggett (1984, p. 185) puts it 'the law relating to mentally disordered offenders is trying to have the best of all worlds. Within the content of a system which is supposed to do justice it is trying to cure those who might be cured and to protect society against those who cannot'.

The problem of the prisons

To paraphrase Barbara Wootton (1959) we may be short of many things in this world but we are not short of offenders. Indeed with a current prison population in England and Wales of over 45 500 (in 1985) increasing all the time, we have – if anything – an abundance, perhaps even a surplus.

The current criminological literature is full of suggestions for reducing that population. There is however little room for manoeuvre. One suggestion is to decriminalise certain types of offences: it has been proposed that drunkeness, for example, ought no longer be a crime. (Drunkeness itself does not lead to imprisonment but failing to pay the fine does, hence the need to decriminalise.) Another suggestion is to prevent courts (and in particular magistrates' courts) from committing civil offenders to prison: that is people who fail to pay maintenance orders, for example, could be dealt with in ways where goods are taken from them and resold with proceeds being sent to the family. Further suggestions are: to take away the powers of courts to send certain offenders to prison, forcing courts to find alternatives; increase parole; to provide an amnesty; and so on and so on.

The mentally disordered offenders could be taken out of the prison system altogether. The 1983 Act provides three opportunities where this can be done: at the remand stage, and at the sentencing and post-sentencing stage. I would like to examine the first and third of these opportunities. At the remand stage, Section 35 of the Act gives powers to courts to remand a person to a hospital for the preparation of a psychiatric report. This is a new power and is based on a recommendation of the Butler Committee (HMSO, 1975, paras 12.1–12.6). Under Section 35 the courts have to be satisfied on the evidence of an approved medical practitioner that there is reason to suppose that the defendant is suffering from one of the four types of mental disorder. The remand can last for a maximum of 12 weeks but cannot be made unless the court is further satisfied that arrangements have been made on the defendant's behalf. The Butler Committee recommended that the courts' power to remand to hospital should not be exercised where a custodial remand is not necessary. The committee expected the first choice of the courts always to be to give bail (para. 12.10). (Incidentally a person remanded under this section is not subject to consent provisions discussed in Chapter 8.)

Section 36 gives power to the Crown court, not the magistrates' courts, to remand an accused suffering from mental illness or severe mental impairment to hospital for treatment for a maximum of 12 weeks. As with Section 35, the defendant must have been charged with an offence which carries imprisonment. Unlike Section 35, Section 36 is restricted to mental illness and severe mental impairment, justified by one commentator on the grounds that 'these forms equate most closely with the medical model of illness and sufferers would be seriously disadvantaged by a long remand in custody whereas those felt to be suffering from psychopathic disorder and mental impairment would not' (quoted in Jones, 1983). I confess the logic of this somehow escapes me. However, Section 48 also gives powers to the Home Secretary for persons suffering from mental illness or severe mental impairment to be removed direct to hospital prior to their sentence. Those powers can only be used when a prisoner's condition is such that immediate removal to a hospital is necessary. Normally, when he is well enough, he is either produced at court or returned to prison to await trial (Jones, 1983).

The Butler Committee justified remands to mental hospitals by contrasting such remands with what it called 'the unhelpful remand to prison' where there were limited facilities for dealing with psychiatric cases. Moreover, under earlier legislation, i.e. the 1959 Act, there were no powers to remand patients to hospitals except through a complicated system whereby bail was granted with a condition of hospital residence. The alternative was a remand to prison (para. 12.2). There was, to be sure, a serious question of the suitability of such a remand but that cannot have been the only reason why the Butler Committee suggested other methods. The possibility of using the mental hospital as a means of reducing the prison population must have been tempting. The committee did not say as much, but perhaps some things are too important and need not be said! Moreover, in practical terms, remands to prison take a disproportionate amount of prison staff time. For example a defendant needs to be admitted formally and discharged formally at the beginning and end of the remand period (or daily if attending court for trial). If he is mentally disordered he may also be additionally troublesome to the prison authorities. To take this type of person out of the prison system offers some relief to the prison authorities disproportionate to the numbers of such offenders.

The third opportunity provided in the Act is to take the mentally disordered offenders out of the prison system at the post-sentence stage.

Under Section 47, the Home Secretary has powers to direct that a person serving a sentence of imprisonment can be removed to or detained in a mental hospital. If the patient recovers before the end of his sentence he can be returned to the prison until his sentence is completed. If he does not recover he is liable to be detained in hospital beyond his date of release. This is not considered to be unjust, as the prisoner would be liable for civil commitment anyway; that he may not see it that way is apparently neither here nor there. The Home Secretary, under Section 50(i)(b) also has powers to release the prisoner on licence 'which would have been exercisable if he had been remitted to such a prison or institution as aforesaid'.

The numbers transferred from prison to mental hospital remain small: 89 in 1971, 70 in 1981 (Hoggett, 1984, p. 181), and bear little or no relation to those said to need hospital treatment. How much these new proposals will affect the prison system is difficult to say but, on past experience, one would expect it to be very little. Prison medical officers in their 6-monthly returns to the Home Office on 30 September 1982 and 31 March 1983 gave a total of 286 and 319 inmates, respectively, said to be sufficiently mentally disordered to warrant transfer. In September 1982 there were 126 sentenced and 160 unsentenced offenders whilst in March 1983 there were 160 sentenced and 159 unsentenced. Surprisingly the trend is downward. In June 1977 for example 769 offenders were identified as requiring mental hospital care and 3 non-criminal or civil prisoners (remember, too, that in 1977 the prison population was lower). What then happens to those identified as mentally disordered who must remain in the prison system? Presumably they wait or are released from prison at the end of their sentence or get better through their own efforts or with the aid of the Prison Medical Service. In 1982 most remained in prison and many had been waiting over a year for transfer (Parliamentary Debates, 6 December 1982, cols 339–40).

These figures provided by the prison medical services of patients being mentally disordered and, by implication, requiring transfer are thought to be on the conservative side. One study put it as high as 20% of the prison population (that would be over 9000 prisoners in the current population), who manifest sufficient psychiatric pathology to warrant attention or intervention. Another put it at 5%, but uses different criteria and talks instead of severe psychiatric disturbance rather than mental disorder. In yet a further study, this time of prisoners remanded into custody, 9% were said to be psychotic (Gostin, 1985). One would have thought therefore that it would have been in the Prison Medical Service's interest to have overplayed the problem. It appears however the prison medical services were using figures calculated on the basis of their experiences and expectations of obtaining a transfer. Many prison medical officers, it seems have stopped recommending all mentally disordered patients for transfer because hospitals will not make places available.

From the prison services' point of view it is clearly desirable that mentally disordered offenders should be given psychiatric treatment or even dealt with elsewhere. It may not be so for the offenders. Once in the psychiatric system, their date of release becomes uncertain, there is always the possibility of being detained for extended periods. Yet, from the prison services' point of view, mentally disordered offenders are occasionally disruptive, often unpredictable and place additional strain on an already overburdened system.

It is not even in accord with traditional theories of punishment that the mentally disordered should justifiably be placed in prison. Retribution, based on deserts, cannot apply; mentally disordered people cannot be said to deserve punishment if they lack the necessary responsibility to be aware of their crime. Similarly, individual deterrence cannot apply; mentally disordered people are not responsible for their actions whilst they remain disordered. Rehabilitation will not apply either, for the prison medical services (as currently constituted) cannot provide the necessary treatment. One would have thought that a simple solution would be to improve existing prison medical services, but this it seems is unlikely. Indeed the Director General of the prison service has said the prison medical service does not purport to offer comprehensive psychiatric treatment because of the belief that transfers of mentally disordered offenders should be made to the National Health Service (in Gostin, 1985). In the meantime, the prisoner presumably waits and waits.

Another solution would be to encourage or require the NHS mental hospitals to take these patients. Here we enter that murky world of professional dominance, mixed with claims and counterclaims relating to the extent of resources, and threats by nursing staff to withdraw labour if transfers are made. Yet, somewhere along the line, the nettle needs to be grasped. It is a problem occuring time and again, whether related to Special Hospitals, Regional Secure Units, or (in this case) transfer from prison. It has beset the prison service since at least 1959 (and the Special Hospitals too for that matter). In spite of lengthy debates on the subject, the solution, is no nearer.

From the prison department's point of view, the argument is clear. Prisons are the only institutions within those two control systems unable to exercise choice about who shall be admitted. Moreover, prisons are inappropriate places to deal with the mentally disordered, and their resources are inadequate anyway. Prisons have therefore to take everyone sent to them yet must rely on the goodwill of others to ease their burdens. Unhappily, say the prison services, other institutions can define their goals and seek appropriate patients, but the prison service cannot. Prisons are grossly overcrowded, mental hospitals much less so. Indeed the ratio of consultants to patients has improved greatly recently, with an aggregate increase in consultants and an aggregate reduction in patients. Given the large numbers of prisoners deemed to be mentally disordered one would have thought a transfer policy was an obvious answer. If the mental hospitals were not prepared to accept such patients then one would have thought they should be compelled to do so.

Not according to the Butler Committee, which put it this way:

We do not think it would be desirable . . . for local psychiatric hospitals to be required to accept mentally disordered offenders provided only that they had a bed available. It is not unreasonable that consultants should establish criteria for selecting patients for treatment, and we have no evidence that in the exercise of their discretion over admission policies consultants in practice act other than in the interests of their staff and other patients.   HMSO (1975) para. 14.7.

It remains unclear why it 'is not unreasonable that consultants should establish criteria for selecting patients for treatment' for that permits health policies to be defined by the consultants. It permits too an approach to medicine which suggests that the key variable is the consultant's definition of his task rather than the needs or medical disabilities of the patients. On the second point (that the Butler Committee 'has no evidence that in their exercise of discretion over admissions . . .'): the evidence, as far as the prison services are concerned is overwhelming. As will be pointed out later in this chapter, so too is the evidence from the Special Hospitals. Moreover, I doubt if any country in the western world other than Britain would allow such professional discretion or would see health policies placed at the discretionary power of a group of senior medical staff. Yet, regrettably, within the prison service we find a similar anomaly making it additionally difficult for others in the prison system to demand a policy of compulsory transfer. Grendon Underwood, the one psychiatric prison in England and Wales, is also permitted to select prisoners for admission. To make matters worse, it can arrange for the transfer of any prisoner who is uncooperative. It uses the model of the mental hospital and, in so doing, it also requires the prisoners to agree to serve their sentences at Grendon. It also refuses to take psychotic prisoners. Visitors to Grendon Underwood may well see, and sometimes are invited to partake in, a great deal of group therapy (the evidence in favour of which is inconclusive and has little or no effect on reconviction rates). But there is nothing for others who cannot sustain such a programme. It is ironic therefore that the prison service which suffers at the hands of the medical professionals produces and preserves those same professional demands.

The Butler Committee concluded their arguments with the following:

Psychiatric hospitals would find it impossible to do their work if they were forced to accommodate all such cases as the courts thought right to send them regardless of their ability to provide suitable treatment. HMSO (1975), para. 14.7.

No evidence was given to support this assertion. Yet, to be fair to the Butler Committee, its arguments are not without substance. One can see how some patients may not fit into the hospitals' treatment plans, that there may not be facilities available, or that psychiatrists may not have the expertise to treat certain patients. Yet the price for accepting that is high: namely, an overcrowded prison system and large numbers of patients left to their own devices. If we really took psychiatrists at their word and accepted their claims to treat the mentally disordered according to their rhetoric I wonder how they then justify this position? And I wonder too what they would say if many mental patients had broken legs, infectious diseases etc. and other physicians refused to have them in their hospitals. It seems one of two conclusions could be drawn: that a similar outrage should be extended to psychiatrists or that psychiatrists claims to be on par with other branches of medicine should be treated with some scepticism. Psychiatrists it seems cannot have it both ways.

It is clear that a serious problem exists surrounding the position of mentally disordered prisoners be it on humanitarian or other grounds. Yet it is not easy to see how the problem can be solved. Consultant psychiatrists, (or, more accurately, the hospital managers acting on the directions of the responsible medical officer), have enjoyed powers to decide their admissions policies since the 1959 Act, and will not easily let them slip away. To do so would, in their view, alter the direction of the mental hospital as a hospital. They fear it would make the mental hospital more akin to the asylums of old whose task it was to contain the criminally mad. Hospitals, in their view, are not places whose duty is to receive and treat those whom the courts think fit. Yet, as was said earlier, the price for that independence is high (in my view, unacceptably high). A solution which encourages rather than compels may be an acceptable compromise, but I doubt if it would work. If not, then more formal measures would be required.

Sentencing the mentally disordered offender

There are provisions in the 1983 Act for offenders to go direct to a hospital under sentence of the court. Section 37 empowers Crown court or a magistrates' court to make a hospital order as an alternative to a penal sentence. It applies to offenders suffering from one of the four specific categories of mental disorder which must be such as to warrant detention in a hospital. The order lasts for a period of 6 months in the first instance, and has the effect as if the patients were committed under Section 3. There are only two significant legal differences between a hospital order and a civil admission for treatment under this Section: the nearest relative of a patient on a hospital order cannot order his discharge under Section 23 and the patient does not have the right to apply to a Mental Health Review Tribunal within 6 months following the hospital order being made. In effect, the first occasion on which a patient on a hospital order or his nearest relative can apply to a tribunal is between 6 and 12 months of the making of the order (Ashworth & Gostin, 1985, p. 219). The courts can make a hospital order in all cases where a person is convicted of an offence punishable with imprisonment unless the sentence is fixed by law (i.e. as in murder). In addition, under Section 41, a court is empowered to add a restriction on the offender's discharge (aimed at protecting the public from serious harm). A restriction order may not be made unless at least one medical practitioner has given oral evidence to the court. Many restricted patients are thought to require the security of a special hospital, admission to which requires the consent of the Home Secretary (Ashworth & Gostin, 1985, p. 221).

What then is the rationale behind hospital orders? The Butler Committee put it this way:

In making a hospital order the court is placing the patient in the hands of the doctors, foregoing (sic) any question of punishment and relinquishing from then onwards its own controls over them. When the doctor or the Mental Health Review Tribunal thinks it right the patient will be discharged. HMSO (1975) para. 14.8.

It is not however as simple as that. First there are retributive questions to consider. The courts can only make a hospital order if 'the offence was punishable with imprisonment'. Yet, having said that, it is also true that hospital orders have been made (and upheld on appeal), where offenders might have served a period of imprisonment less than that of the hospital order. The justice of this remains unclear and less so when (on appeal) hospital orders have been substituted by a period of imprisonment. Then there is the problem of the mentally handicapped. The Butler Committee was concerned about placing the mentally handicapped on a hospital order because of the possible injustice created, fearing that they might spend longer in hospital than they would have done in prison. Yet at the other extreme, offenders convicted of serious offences have been placed on a hospital order, and discharged by the hospital after a short time (presumably because their mental disorder was less severe than considered earlier, or the mental disorder responded to treatment or – for some reason or other – the hospital was not prepared to keep the offender any longer). In these cases, such offenders may have avoided a rather lengthy custodial sentence. There is also the possibility of offenders being placed on civil commitment orders under Section 3 when the hospital order has expired , which they may see as less than just.

On the matter of injustice, there is special provision under Section 37(3) which applies only to magistrates' courts where a court 'if satisfied that the accused did the act or made the omission charged the court may if it thinks fit, make such an order without convicting him'. The court need hear nothing more than the evidence of arrest. The defendant does not plead, or call witnesses. This provision, which is as near as one can get to providing magistrates' courts with powers similar to those in the Crown courts for 'unfit to plead' cases turn out to be a convenient way of allowing magistrates courts to circumvent complex legal and jurisprudential problems. To complicate matters further, the law does not require a link to be made between the offender's mental condition and the crime. A hospital order can be made therefore when there is no direct causal connection between the mental condition and the current offence. Indeed an offender may develop a mental disorder some time after the crime was committed and still be subject to a hospital order, if he is disordered when he appears at court. In these circumstances, the court appears to operate as if it were adjourning proceedings *sine die* and making the hospital order as if it were making an order under Section 3 (the treatment order). The offence in this case is of secondary importance except that it must carry the possibility of imprisonment. Thus we have created two types of sentence and, I would add, numerous uncertainties and ambiguities to go with it. We are, I think, entitled to know also whether the offence is important or not, and if so whether the courts should establish links between the mental disorder and the crime. As things stand at present, the whole business is plagued with problems because the law is trying to meet too many competing demands or wanting the best of all possible worlds.

Taking a wider view and passing over questions of injustice there is no clear statement as to why some offenders are selected for a hospital order, given the large number of offenders deemed to be mildly disordered at the time of sentence. Probation officers see some offenders and advise the courts accordingly but, even then, only a small number of offenders would see a probation officer before sentence – particularly in busy London and provincial courts. As with so much else in the penal system, the offender's previous record seems to be the important component. An earlier admission to a mental hospital is likely to alert courts to the possibility of current mental disorder.

Powers given to the Crown courts to 'make restrictions' on the time spent in hospital add a further twist to the list of complexities. The problem is the peculiar manner in which the courts have interpreted the law. Restrictions may be imposed for a definite period or without limit of time (Section 41(1)). If the restriction ends whilst the patient is still in hospital, he becomes a patient on an ordinary hospital order and is dealt with accordingly. Relatively few patients are placed on order with time limits (about 3% of all hospital orders in 1978, and 10% in 1982), for it is argued there is no means of knowing in advance when recovery can be predicted. Yet, without a time limit, the patient is virtually on a life sentence. The patient cannot be discharged, transferred to another hospital or given leave of absence without the Home Secretary's consent. Gostin views this sentence with alarm, arguing that special restrictions ought not to last longer than a period proportionate to the gravity of the offence for which they were imposed – at least unless the case meets the criteria which would justify the imposition of life imprisonment on a person not suffering from a treatable mental disorder. (Ashworth & Gostin, 1985, p. 224).

The 1983 Act has made two changes aimed at reforming the restriction order; granting patients automatic reviews to Mental Health Review Tribunals (MHRT) and imposing additional qualifications to limit their use. In the first, and largely as a result of a decision by the European Court (*X* v. United Kingdom 1981) restricted patients have a right of application to a MHRT. Section 41(6) also requires the responsible medical officer to examine the patient at such intervals, not exceeding 1 year and report accordingly to the Secretary of State. Interestingly enough MHRTs dealing with restricted patients must be chaired by a circuit judge or recorder and, like all patients appearing before a MHRT, can be legally represented. One would have thought that on the face of it this was a considerable advance. Ashworth & Gostin (1985, p. 224) however raise doubts. They say the tribunal has a duty to discharge a restricted patient if the disorder is no longer 'of a degree which makes it appropriate for him to be detained in a hospital for medical treatment', and 'it is not necessary for the health and safety of other persons that he should receive such treatment'. Yet to be placed on a restriction order the patient had to be adjudged as being capable of causing serious harm – or, in other words, the criteria for discharge are different and more narrow than for admission. This, say Ashworth & Gostin (1985, p. 225) is misconceived.

There is also the question of the use of the restriction order by the courts. Here sentencing practices become tied up with questions relating to dangerousness, and, once again, professional dominance. The 1983 Act under Section 41(1) required the court to state that special restrictions 'were necessary for the protection of the public from serious harm'. To arrive at this conclusion the court should 'have regard to the nature of the offence, the antecedents of the offender and the risk of his committing further offences if set at large'. A restriction order is protective and the court's decision predictive.

The justification for including 'serious harm' was to narrow the types of offence from which the public required protection. Under the 1959 Act the court could impose a restriction order where '. . . it appears to the court, having regard to the nature of the offence, the antecedents of the offender and the risk of committing further offences if set at large, that it is necessary for the protection of the public so to do . . .'. That Act gave no indication of the seriousness of the offences from which the public was intended to be protected. The result was frequent misuse of the order where petty recidivists and the like were swept into the system because of the strong probability that they would persist with similar offences in the future.

For this the courts were largely to blame. Yet, unhappily, the problem has not been confined to sentencing the mentally disordered but extends to other types of offenders. Under the 1948 Criminal Justice Acts two such similar protective sentences were available; corrective training for offenders under the age of 30 and preventative detention for older ones. These sentences were repealed under the 1967 Criminal Law Act after widespread criticisms. It was noted that sentences of preventative detention were often passed on offenders who had committed relatively minor crimes (i.e. theft of less than £5.00) and were justified by the courts on the basis of the offenders' past records. Corrective training was similarly used. The message was and is clear: whenever protective sentences are introduced the courts tend to use them to deal with social nuisances rather than serious offenders. Protective sentences become a form of social defence to be used against the feckless and inadequate.

It is difficult to explain why this should be so. No one denies the problem facing courts when presented with highly recidivistic offenders (often petty, but not always so) who reappear in spite of every attempt to change their criminal natures. Yet it is almost as if the courts see these types of sentences granting them a lifeline, and more so if a psychiatric diagnosis can be attached to an offender and a hospital willing to accept him. Restriction orders have similarly been used in the past. Some mentally handicapped offenders have been placed on restriction orders for relatively minor offences, perhaps offences on indecency or the like. Of course some mentally handicapped are very persistent offenders and the temptation must be great to 'protect the public' from them. The cost of doing so is, however, high. In financial terms, if the offender goes to a Special Hospital as he sometimes does, it costs £30,000 per year or about £600 per week to keep him there (HMSO, 1985). In social and moral terms, the cost is more difficult to calculate yet probably also high. It remains to be seen if the new legislation will produce a more considered approach. Bearing in mind the court's track record, I admit to being sceptical.

Then there is the predictive aspect to the sentence. To protect from serious harm is to imply *inter alia* that the offender is dangerous. Yet dangerousness remains an elusive concept (Bowden, 1985). Dangerousness is not a medical or psychiatric quality discoverable by clinicians, but a social concept dependent on the situation in which the offender finds himself. Bowden (1985, p. 277), in an otherwise well-argued paper, nonetheless sees the psychiatrist's role as central in identifying the dangerous, arguing that it 'suits the institutions of society to allow the psychiatrist to practice in the field of dangerousness because he can be relied upon to act conservatively in his deliberations'. This is not so: it has been psychiatrists who – more often than not – have wanted to practise in the field and (far from acting conservatively) they tend, if anything, to overpredict. With overprediction there is, paradoxically, a greater level of certainty. Those patients who become false positives cannot show that the predictions about them were wrong for they remain incarcerated. In contrast, false negatives (that is, those not predicted to commit offences yet who did so nonetheless) bring forth increasing demands for harsher sentences.

I do not wish to enter the current debate on dangerousness, for that would take us into a much wider set of arguments. If however attention is confined to the restriction order there seems to be an assumption that dangerousness and certain types of mental disorders are linked. They may well be, but it is not always easy to decide on the nature of that link. There are three possibilities. First that a patient may be dangerous and mentally disordered yet, when cured of his disorder, he may nonetheless remain dangerous. Second, the patient may remain mentally disordered but, over time, cease to be dangerous. And third, the patient may continue to be mentally disordered and continue to be dangerous or, conversely, cease to be mentally disordered and likewise cease to be dangerous. The 1983 Act does not, nor could it ever, help judges or courts make such fine predictions yet it does appear to foster the notion that the third of these possibilities is the only one worth considering. Much psychiatric practice also fosters that assumption for the nature of psychiatric explanation makes plausible connections between mental disorder and dangerousness when psychiatrists produce their biography of the patient.

There is also the interesting question about whether restriction orders are required in the first place. The conventional answer would be I suppose that some people are sufficiently disordered and dangerous to require protective sentencing. But they are not the only dangerous people in our society. Many others, including those causing death by reckless driving and neglectful employers who cause industrial accidents produce great harm and many more deaths than the type of patient considered appropriate to be sentenced to a restriction order. The difference according to some commentators (quoted in Bowden, 1985) is that the mentally disordered offender remains outside or apart from the functionally acceptable process central to our daily lives. The motor car, the factory etc. are intrinsic to our social order. The mentally abnormal dangerous offender produces unpredictable and uncontrollable behaviour offering a dysfunctional alternative. One can see a sort of sociological logic about the answer but can we I wonder let the matter rest there. Certainly we ought to ask more searching questions about the morality of protective sentences but so too did we ought to ask questions about other dangerous people in our society, whatever their function or dysfunction to society as a whole. If restrictions are required for one group then some such similar controls ought to be further imposed on the other.

I have no wish to deny that mentally disordered offenders involved in offences classified as serious and harmful ought not to be detained. That however is not the problem. The problem is about the nature and extent of the sentence. Yet the simplest answer to many of the questions posed above would I think be to sentence on the basis of proportionality or retribution. If, at the end of the sentence, the offender was still deemed to be mentally disordered then he would qualify for civil commitment like anyone else. Such a proposal would avoid all heart-searching questions relating to dangerousness, to prediction, to restriction orders, even to debates about the link between mental disorder and crime. It would also resurrect arguments about justice which become submerged under a welter of other arguments, most of which are tangential to the main questions. Sometimes I think we make it hard for ourselves and our offenders by trying to achieve more than can reasonably be expected. A return to a less complicated method understood by all, including the courts, would, I think, improve things.

Some problems relating to the special hospitals

The Secretary of State for Social Services has a duty under Section 4 of the National Health Service Act 1977 to 'provide and maintain establishments

. . . for persons subject to detention under the Mental Health Act 1983 who in his opinion require treatment on account of their dangerousness, violent or criminal propensities'. Section 4 of the 1977 Act replaced Section 97 of the Mental Health Act 1959. The Special Hospitals (Rampton, Broadmoor, Park Lane, and Moss Side in England and Wales, and Carstairs in Scotland) are under the direct control and management of the Secretary of State. The control of these Special Hospitals was recently criticised by an All Party Select Committee on Social Services as being in need of better management and more accountability (HMSO, 1985). Existing, as they do, outside the NHS administrative system. Nonetheless under Section 123 of the 1983 Act, the Secretary of State has powers to transfer patients from a Special Hospital to an ordinary mental hospital). Interestingly enough under Section 123(2) 'the Secretary of State may give directions for the transfer of any patient who is for the time being liable to be so detained into a hospital which is not a special hospital'. At the time of writing (1985) no such direction has yet been given.

In Special Hospitals often the responsible medical officer (when he considers that a patient no longer requires treatment in conditions of security in a special hospital and in the case of a non-restricted patient) discharges patients to a NHS hospital. In the case of a restricted patient, his duty is to recommend to the Home Secretary his conditional discharge or transfer. (Hamilton, 1985, p. 117). About two-thirds of releases are by transfer. The number leaving Special Hospitals was 203 for 1982 as against 222 for the previous year. On 31 December 1983 there was a total of 1686 patients in the four Special Hospitals in England and Wales, of whom 553 were restricted patients and 1133 unrestricted. 58% were classified as suffering from mental illness, 24% psychopathic disorder, 10% mental impairment and 7% severe mental impairment (Hamilton, 1985, p. 108).

All countries require Special Hospitals, although not necessarily called by that name. That is there needs to be a place at the end of the line, a residual institution taking the most severe patients and detaining them in conditions of maximum security. Some countries separate the criminal and the civil, others as in Britain provide institutions which tackle both. Being institutions of last resort, those who manage them have always to face two important questions: which patients are to go in, and (once in) when and where do the patients go on discharge? In Britain, decisions to admit and discharge from the Special Hospitals are taken by the Secretary of State, supported by medical recommendations from specially qualified psychiatrists. Admission is often by way of the courts but may be from ordinary mental hospitals. The medical recommendations are obviously crucial to the whole process. Gostin (1985) however, believes there are many instances where NHS psychiatrists exaggerate the patient's condition to produce the necessary transfer. Be that as it may, once in there is the problem of how to get the patients out.

As matters stand at present, discharge is likely to be to an NHS hospital where security is less strict, the atmosphere more relaxed, and adjustment can take place in conditions more akin to the outside world. Recently out of 203 discharged from Special Hospital, 132 were transferred to other NHS hospitals. The NHS hospitals become a halfway house where, if the patient is able to adjust, he can move out of the hospital system altogether; if unable to adjust he can be returned to the Special Hospital. To assist transfers to the mental hospitals, the DHSS has agreed that it will give an unconditional undertaking to re-admit a patient if, within the first few months after transfer, the patient does not settle, thus providing a sort of trial period (Hamilton, 1985).

How to get out: that remains the problem. Here again we make it hard for ourselves, or rather for the patients. Dell (1980) showed that one in three of patients were awaiting transfer out of the Special Hospitals, and had been waiting for over 2 years compared with one in ten, 3 years previously. There were 183 patients awaiting transfer for whom no NHS hospital bed could be found. In addition, many more patients were suitable for transfer but were not being recommended because there was little or no chance of the recommendations being accepted. Since that time the position has, if anything, worsened. There were, at 31 December 1983, 223 patients awaiting transfer of whom 21 had been waiting over 3 years. The percentage awaiting transfer has gone up from 9.9% in 1979, when Dell conducted her research, to 10.3% in 1982 and higher in 1983 (Hamilton, 1985, p. 120). In July 1984, 16 patients had been waiting over 4 years (Parliamentary Debates, 23 July 1984, cols 416–37).

To some extent, the Special Hospitals themselves cannot remain free from criticisms although they say they operate under very difficult circumstances. Frequent changes of staff disrupt continuity and restrict the ability to get to know patients and promote their cases. Then there is the quality of the staff (psychiatric, nursing or otherwise). It is not necessary to go over old ground here and resurrect those recent enquiries into the staff at some Special Hospitals. Whilst it is unrealistic to expect uniformly high standards, staff who are less than satisfactory in institutions such as Special Hospitals regrettably make existing defects more glaring. Where records are not updated, patients seen infrequently, and medications not kept under tight review it is hardly surprising that the welfare of patients appears not to be of primary consideration.

The problem is in part one which stems from the policies of the NHS hospitals and their reluctance to take patients from the Special Hospitals. Having pursued an 'open-door' policy for a number of years, and certainly, since the 1959 Act, NHS hospitals claim they have few facilities for the treatment of potentially disruptive patients. This 'open-door' policy has been generally beneficial, no one denies that, but mental hospitals have rarely been completely 'open-door'. Most retain some locked wards and most offer some form of security, in addition to the Regional Secure Units, to be examined later in this chapter. It is suggested that they could take patients if they so wanted and suggested too that most have facilities to do so. Why then do they not?

Whether by accident or design assistance for the NHS hospitals has come in the form of Trade Union action. COHSE, with many psychiatric nurses as members, have taken industrial action and refuses to admit certain mentally disordered offenders from the Special Hospitals, as well as from the Courts. After one celebrated case (Regina v. Brazil from Bristol Crown Court) when COHSE refused the patient admission without, I would add, having seen the patient beforehand, the National Executive of the union issued the following directive.

That nurses should be able to choose whether they want to work with or near abnormal offenders in mental hospitals if they consider safety and security provisions are not adequate . . . This decision will continue until the union is satisfied that the level of the treatment facilities do not expose nursing staff to unacceptable degrees of bodily danger.   Quoted in Gostin, (1985).

This decision has never been reversed and industrial action has continued. (Whether this could be construed as being against Section 129 of the 1983 Act which says 'Any person who without reasonable cause otherwise obstructs any such person in the exercise of his functions shall be guilty of an offence' remains to be seen.) In 1976 the DHSS issued a circular in an attempt to reduce the anxieties of hospital staff concerning the management of violent or potentially violent patients (DHSS, 1976). COHSE instructed its members to ignore the DHSS guidelines and subsequently issued its own. This led to the celebrated Ashingdene case. Ashingdene was a patient at Broadmoor Hospital who was recommended for transfer to a hospital in Kent by an MHRT with the support of his consultant, and confirmed by the Secretary of State. Oakwood hospital in Kent was prepared to accept him. COHSE members opposed the move and threatened industrial action. MIND and others brought the case to the European Court and argued that Ashingdene was detained unlawfully and in more secure accommodation than was necessary. The court action was unsuccessful but, even so, illustrates the desperate positions in which some patients find themselves. Of course nursing staff deal with the day-to-day affairs of patients and one has some sympathy with their position but I agree with Gostin when he says

in seeking to obtain more support and a fair share of resources nurses should not deprive patients of their basic rights to treatment in the least restrictive setting possible.   Gostin (1985)

During the debates on the 1983 Act, Parliament attempted to resolve the problem of professional discretion which is at the heart of the matter. At the Special Standing Committee on the Bill an amendment was introduced which stated

The Secretary of State shall make regulations concerning the consultations which shall be undertaken by the managers of a hospital in considering the arrangements to be made for the admission of the offender to that hospital in the event of such an order being made. . . .   10 June 1982, amendment No. 118.

The amendment resulted in a tied vote, the chairman declaring himself with the 'Noes' and the amendment lost. In the debate itself both sides of the argument were presented. Those in favour wanted legislation 'to concentrate the minds of those who have the responsibility' (Parliamentary Debates Special Standing Committee, 10 June 1982, Col. 495), those against because they 'did not believe that it will be easy to overcome medical reluctance by statutory means because we are dealing with clinical judgments . . . What we can do is improve knowledge by more cooperation and more education (ibid, col. 506). I remain pessimistic about the outcome, for there is little to suggest much will change and much to suggest the problem will get worse. If one takes the number of hospital orders alone as an indication of hospitals being prepared to accept similar patients, the trend is clear. In 1966 there were 1440 hospital orders, in 1976 there were 924, in 1979 there were 506 and by the 1980s the numbers were continuing to fall (ibid, col. 495). By the same argument, I cannot see much change occuring in the transfers of patients from the Special Hospitals. Other countries may look askance at this peculiarly British problem, being unable to appreciate the relative impotence of the courts and the relative potency of the medical profession and the Trade Unions.

Regional Secure Units

Regional Secure Units (RSUs) were to ease the overcrowding in the prisons by taking mentally disordered offenders already under sentence, and take pre-sentenced offenders direct from the courts. They were intended also to reduce the numbers of remand prisoners. They would also take patients from the Special Hospitals who required less than maximum security. Yet, far from being a salvation, they have made very little difference to the overall set of problems. In fact they are expensive to run, and produce a middle tier in the security system without reducing many of the problems which beset the existing system.

RSUs stemmed directly from the report of Butler Committee or rather the interim report of that committee. Their origins can be traced to 1959, through to 1961 (under a working party set up by Enoch Powell), and to the Glancy Report. In 1974 the then Secretary of State for Social Services (Barbara Castle) accepted the recommendations of the Glancy and Butler Committees, the latter seeing the development of RSUs as a matter of urgency to relieve overcrowding in the Special Hospitals. The Butler Committee wanted 2000 places for patients in secure units. This figure of 2000 is incidentally subject to considerable variation; sometimes there is talk of 1000 (as in the Glancy Report), sometimes even less than that. It is expected that there will be about 700 places available by the end of 1986 designed, according to the DHSS, for 'patients who are continuously behaviourally disturbed or who are persistently violent or considered a danger to the public, albeit not an immediate one' (1975).

The sentiments behind the development of RSUs (or NHS Secure Treatment Units, as COHSE wishes to call them,) are laudable. To repeat the point: they are intended to reduce overcrowding in the Special Hospitals, to remove some patients from the Special Hospitals who did not need that type of secure conditions, to reduce the number of mentally ill in the prisons (for obvious and varied reasons), and to develop forensic psychiatric services for the courts. All these reasons seem to warrant general support. Were RSUs in fact the best way to deal with these areas? They provide semi-secure provision within the ordinary mental hospital. One factor to consider is that RSUs must imply that the open-door policy, so lauded by psychiatrists and mental health officials for four decades, is almost over (or, if not almost over, then can be applied at medical discretion). The open-door policy was always a statement of intent rather than anything else. Yet, whilst it remained, there was at least the strong possibility that fewer locked wards would exist and more hospitals would see the open-door policy as desirable. I suspect, but do not know, that RSUs might unwittingly reverse that policy by giving credibility once more to formal types of security and restraint. Certainly when RSUs were mooted and discussed in earnest in 1975–6, some hospitals refused to consider them believing that they would damage their progressive image. I think they were right to see it that way. There may be and probably is justification for some secure accommodation within mental hospitals, if transfers are to be accepted from the Special Hospitals and elsewhere. The problem is that these secure units look surprisingly like mini-Special Hospitals, staffed by personnel directed towards forensic psychiatry and with increased perimeter security. Their designation and physical separation from the main hospital make them targets for all types of grievances and fears (eg. grievances that a group of mentally disordered patients attract financial support in contrast to the cutbacks in spending elsewhere, thereby depriving others who seem to be more deserving from such benefits – the staff ratio is expected to be 1 – and fears that units with high perimeter security will be used as punishment blocks for the unworthy). There are also fears that Regional Health Authorities may try to save running costs, cut back on staff ratios and force the units to use more obvious forms of security and physical restraint.

Unhappily the history and development of RSUs bode ill for the future. First there is the problem of the missing money. Between 1976 and 1982 over £26 million were directly allocated for secure provision for the mentally disordered. This was not spent for that purpose, by some Regional Health Authorities. It was diverted elsewhere. On a crude calculation, the £26 million allocated to produce 700 beds by 1986 means a cost of about £400 000 per bed. Moreover, whatever one may think of RSUs, the manner in which this large amount of money was spent must lead one to ask what sort of system is this which provides money on such a scale, and finds it is diverted elswhere? What improvements could have been made in other services if £26 million had been spent on the Special Hospitals, the Prison Medical Services or mental hospitals generally?

There is also the question of the patients for the RSUs. It comes as no surprise to see, although I remain saddened at the figures, that over one-third of all first admissions to RSUs come from local hospitals. (Indeed, the RSU I know best has a higher percentage than this.) Assume that this trend will remain constant, of the 700 beds available one-third will be used by the local hospitals, leaving about 460 to be used elsewhere, i.e. the Special Hospitals, the Courts and the prisons. Given that the reasons for developing RSUs in the first place was to reduce the numbers of patients in the Special Hospitals and prisons, it is saddening that these patients stand little chance of being so transferred. Already (1985) there are complaints from prison medical officers who are finding it difficult to get patients transferred to RSUs, and complaints too from the Special Hospitals for similar reasons.

Yet RSUs force us again to re-examine one of the perennial problems in psychiatry; that is the distinction between the acute and the chronic patients. Always it seems the chronic are less favoured, for the chronic do not fit into the psychiatrists self-image of a doctor who is essentially a diagnostician who provides relief from illness through treatment. Yet it is the chronic patient who often needs to be taken out of the Special Hospitals and out of the prisons. It does not seem that they go to the RSUs. Why do they not? The answer is, presumably, because chronic patients would become long-stay patients, thereby making RSUs identical to the Special Hospitals. Yet, if RSUs are to offer that least restrictive environment which everyone agrees is desirable, it is from the Special Hospitals and prisons that these patients should come.

The argument about RSUs needs to be attacked at its roots. I am suggesting that the concept of RSUs was misconstrued. The haste, bordering on panic i.e. the manner in which they were introduced, and the manner in which they have provided a second tier of secure provision, and the type of patients they have taken – not I would add with any suggestion that the type of treatments given will be qualitatively superior to that provided elsewhere – does not, I think, meet the problems of the Special Hospitals or prisons. That can only be met by a requirement which places obligations on the mental hospitals to receive certain types of patients. That will not come through the development of any additional secure units. We return again to the problem of professional dominance and all that entails.

Conclusion

The problems of the mentally abnormal offender remain as entrenched as ever. First there are the problems related to the aims of sentencing: what are we trying to do? If we are trying for 'the best of all possible worlds' ought we not to recognise that mixing penal and treatment philosophies tends to produce only a large element of confusion. I have suggested throughout this chapter that wherever possible a return to retributive sentencing may help ease, if not solve, some of the problems. Also there is the problem of patients in prisons or Special Hospitals who, for one reason or another, are inappropriately placed. I have suggested that professional dominance helps produce unfavourable situations, that the nettle ought to be grasped and the powers of those able to obstruct should be reduced. Whatever some might say measures which encourage professionals rather than control them will, I am sure be less successful. The 1983 Act has not, on these counts, done much to solve such problems although in some respects it has made a small number of worthwhile changes.

There can be few other areas of mental health legislation which are as intractable as those concerned with the mentally abnormal offender. In 1975 the Butler Committee reported (HMSO, 1975), with specific reference to the Mentally Abnormal offender. In the areas covered by this chapter that report did little; unless one takes a less critical view of RSUs than that adopted here. It is unlikely that there will be another such report within the next decade. In my view, the Butler Committee represents another lost opportunity.

I do not wish to convey that there are solutions, short term or otherwise, though there are some arguments more favourable than others within the current context. The solutions that we seek will depend on our priorities. If we think more patients in Special Hospitals ought to be given opportunities to live in less restricted environments and if we view mentally disordered prisoners in a similar light then we need to deal with the admission procedures of the mental hospitals. If we see RSUs largely as an irrelevance to these questions, then we shall or ought to be more insistent in our demands. If too we see ambiguities and confusion about making hospital orders then we shall proceed accordingly. If we do all that we shall have done much.

The long-term solutions are no less difficult. I have mentioned the quality of staff in the Special Hospitals, perhaps unfairly singling them out for attention. There is no point in labouring the problems of Rampton graphically described in the Boynton Report (DHSS, 1980) but many such problems persist nevertheless (not just amongst the nursing staff). There have been improvements, to be sure, but there is still some way to go. It is regrettable therefore that MHRTs do not have, as part of their brief, a mechanism for drawing formal attention to perceived abuses of patients' rights. MHRTs are often in a privileged position to see more than most about what is going on. Other long-term solutions relate to the discharge of mentally abnormal offenders and, of course, that link with community care.

This chapter has emphasised professional dominance and I have tried to show that one barrier is the power we give to some professionals to permit them to define the priorities in mental health care. I would hope that by removing that barrier some immediate problems could be eased.

CHAPTER 7

The discharge of patients from institutions

Elaborate mechanisms and procedures have been created to deal with the admission of patients to mental hospitals but few concerned with their discharge. Offender patients or patients admitted on Sections 2, 3 or 4 find more often than not that the order ends, without ceremony, and they remain in hospitals as voluntary patients or are discharged. The former is more likely if they are on short-term orders; the average length of admission being about 3 months. Informal patients are similarly discharged as and when the registered medical practitioner deems it appropriate.

Types of discharge

To concentrate first on the formal patients: Section 23 grants powers to the MRO, the hospital managers and the nearest relatives to discharge or apply for discharge of formal patients. For patients on a short-term order, powers of early discharge are used infrequently by the responsible medical officer, slightly more so for those on a 6 months treatment order. But even so, it is interesting to observe that there are no legal criteria for determining discharge; again it is all a matter for clinical judgment. Nor is the medical practitioner obliged to discharge a patient if the criteria used at the admission stage are no longer fulfilled. There are secondary tacit assumptions that patients will be granted discharge as soon as they are ready, with, the further assumption that the hospital will return patients to the community as quickly as possible. This is perhaps so, for few hospitals would wish to detain patients who had no reason to remain there.

The second form of discharge is for the patient to abscond. The term 'abscond' covers two distinct areas in the legislation; the first where the patient is in legal custody, that is he is required or authorised by, or under the Act to be conveyed to any place, or be kept in custody or be detained in a place of safety (Section 137(1)). Patients who abscond from legal custody can be detained by certain authorised personnel, social workers etc. who in so doing have 'all the powers authorities protection and privileges which a constable has within the area for which he acts as a constable' (Section 137(2)) (This legal point incidentally tends to make some social workers uneasy for they wish to avoid being seen equivalent to a constable. In their enthusiasm to help patients, they try to distance themselves from those in formal authority.) There are curious provisions in Section 137 whereby patients absconding from legal custody can only be taken within certain time limits; for those in a place of safety within 72 hours of arrival at the place of safety, for those on an emergency order under Section 4 within 24 hours and for those on other forms of civil commitment within 14 days (Section 138(3)).

The other use of the term 'abscond' is when the patient leaves a hospital to which he has been compulsorily admitted, or where he is required to live by a guardian, or fails to return at the end of leave of absence or breaks a residence condition in his leave of absence. In these cases the following conditions apply:

an in-patient detained for 6 or 72 hours under Section 5 or a patient admitted for assessment for 72 hours or 28 days can never be re-taken once that term has gone by (Section 18(5)). Patients admitted for treatment can only be recaptured within 28 days which begin on the first day of absent without leave. If a patient is not taken in this time the authority to detain him ends automatically (Section 18(4)).

This 28 day limit applies equally to ordinary hospital order patients but restricted patients can be recaptured at any time (Hoggett, 1984, p. 233)

These rather quaint provisions hark back to the nineteenth century and particularly to the 1890 Lunacy Act. Absconding patients were allowed to remain free if they were able to avoid capture for a given period (this being sufficient to assume they were competent to look after themselves). It is not clear why such provisions should remain in contemporary legislation. Firstly, there exists an open-door policy in mental hospitals, unlike the tight security offered hitherto. Escape is no longer difficult. Secondly, modern hospitals make little or no attempt to recapture absconders – again unlike their nineteenth century counterparts. Thirdly, the assumption that absconders are demonstrating a capacity to look after themselves should they remain free for a given period seems unrealistic. They may be protected and cared for by family and friends. It is bad enough that these provisions should exist for detained civil patients but are without justification whatsoever for offenders 'to discharge themselves by operation of the law', it adds little to the mental hospitals' credulity, and much to the existing confusion relating to the mentally abnormal offender. The Butler Committee recommended that 'these crude safeguards' be abolished, the more so with the introduction of Mental Health Review Tribunals (HMSO, 1975, para. 14.15). Its advice was not accepted.

The third form of discharge is when the hospital grants the patient leave of absence. (There are others, and for a more detailed discussion, see Hoggett, 1984). This form is in some ways the most interesting and it leads directly towards a discussion on aftercare. For, under Section 17(1), leave of absence can be granted by the responsible medical officer to any compulsory patient. If the patient is a restricted one, then the Home Secretary's permission is required. Otherwise this section applies to all detained patients including those on a hospital order or a guardianship order. Leave can be for a specified period for a specified occasion or for the remainder of the order. Where appropriate, further leave can be granted at the direction of the responsible medical officer without recalling the patient to hospital. The responsible medical officer can insist on conditions; these could include staying in another hospital, living with a particular person, or attending elsewhere for treatment. Under Section 17(5), patients cannot be recalled to hospital if their period of detention has lapsed or they have had 6 months' continuous leave, unless the patient was absent without leave at the end of the period. Consent to treatment regulations apply to the patient during his period of leave. (Jones, 1984)

The Butler Committee saw the home leave provisions as 'very sensible' and hoped in the future that home leave would be more widely used as a prelude to discharge or as a stage in the process of discharge (HMSO, 1975, para. 7.3). The committee thought it would help with aftercare arrangements, for the committee regarded aftercare as a valuable aid for discharged patients. In this it followed the Percy Commission, which were similarly enthusiastic wanting aftercare taken over by the social services departments rather than the hospital authorities. The result under the 1983 Act, was a compromise. After much parliamentary debate, and largely due to the insistence of the House of Lords, aftercare provisions of a more specific nature were enacted. They are under Section 117 which says:

It shall be the duty of the District Health Authority and of the local Social Services Authority to provide . . . after care services for any person to whom this section applies until such time as the District Health Authority and the local social services authority are satisfied that the person concerned is no longer in need of such services.

Section 117(2).

These provisions apply to patients on a treatment order, i.e. Section 3, and on a hospital order i.e. Section 37, and patients transferred to hospital under Sections 47 and 48.

The Government was opposed to Section 117, arguing that such aftercare provisions were unnecessary, for under the National Health Services Act there existed powers to provide aftercare facilities for patients suffering from all forms of illness. Mental disorders would be so included. Others saw this as inadequate. They wanted legal provisions which placed a duty on local authorities to consider the aftercare needs of each patient, and specifically the mentally disordered. Gostin (1983, p. 73) regards even this as inadequate. He argues that it would have been preferable had the Act imposed a duty to provide aftercare for all patients detained or not. He says 'the act should also have made clear what services are required: the term after care is left undefined'.

The next and probably the most important form of discharge is through the MHRTs. These stemmed from the Percy Commission which considered that patients may wish to seek justification for the use of compulsory powers through some independent body. In its view the

only satisfactory arrangement would be for the justification for the patients detention in hospital or control under guardianship to be reviewed by some local body which could itself re-assess the case from both medical and non-medical points of view. We therefore recommend that patients should have an opportunity to apply to a tribunal which would consist of medical and non-medical members selected from a panel of suitable persons for each hospital region.   HMSO (1957) para. 442.

The commission believed that MHRTs were superior to other forms of appeal procedures, whether to the managers of the local hospital (who would appear to the patient to be biassed), or the justices (who would have to rely on medical evidence and who would tend to operate as a court with all the resulting stigma attached), or through an independent medical opinion, or through boards of visitors, or through the scrutiny of documents by the Board of Control. The commission thought that the success of any MHRT system would depend very largely on the experience and calibre of the members of the tribunals, and in particular of the regional chairman (HMSO, 1957, para. 454). Indeed, it does although – as some commentators have pointed out – the structure of the tribunal is probably as important (Fennel, 1977; Peay, 1982.).

MHRTs were established under the 1959 Act and have been retained and strengthened under the 1983 Act. They are independent bodies whose duty it is to hear applications and references by or in respect of patients detained or subject to guardianship. As presently constituted, tribunal members are drawn from panels of lawyers, medical practitioners and lay people with appropriate experience in administration or social services. During the parliamentary debates on the 1983 Act, there was a fear that courts lack confidence in MHRTs as a means of protecting the public interest and courts might be reluctant therefore to make hospital orders for serious offender patients. Accordingly, the Act requires that where a patient is subject to a restriction order the president of the MHRTs will normally be a circuit judge but could also be a recorder (see also Gostin, 1983 p. 41). The constitution and powers of MHRTs are dealt with in Part *V* of the 1983 Act, covering Sections 65–79.

Section 66 provides details and identifies the occasions on which a patient or his nearest relative may make an application to a tribunal. Briefly and to avoid entering into too many legal details there are eight major features (for a more comprehensive review see Gostin, Rassaby & Buchan, 1984; Hoggett, 1984). Under Section 66 of the 1983 Act, applications may be made by:

(i)   a patient is admitted to hospital for assessment under Section 2 (the patient may apply within 14 days of admission);

(ii)   a patient is admitted to hospital for treatment under Section 3 (the patient may apply within 6 months of admission);

(iii)   a patient is received into guardianship under Section 7 (the patient may apply within 6 months of the date of the order);

(iv)   a report is furnished under Section 16; that is where the patient is to have his diagnosis reclassified (a patient or nearest relative may apply within 28 days of the date they were informed of the reclassification);

(v)   a patient is transferred from guardianship under Section 19 (the patient may apply within 6 months of the date of transfer);

(vi)   a report is furnished under Section 20; that is where a patient detained for treatment or under guardianship is further detained (the patient may apply within each period following renewal of the order; that is in the first 6 months following renewal and in each subsequent 12 months);

(vii)   a report is furnished under Section 25; that is where the nearest relative is restricted from making an application for the patients discharge (the nearest relative who has requested discharge of the patient may apply within 28 days of being told that the responsible medical officer has prevented that discharge);

(viii)   an order is made under Section 29; that is where a nearest relative of a patient detained in hospital or subject to a guardianship order has had his authority removed by a County court (he may apply to an MHRT once every 12 months).

For these purposes, one application can be made during the specified period. Withdrawn applications do not count. The eight listed features are not exhaustive, others relate to reception orders under the old Lunacy Acts, from prison to hospital (for a full list see Gostin *et al*, 1984 pp. 44–8) although those given above are for these purposes the most important. (They also cover matters relating to other chapters in this volume, notably: guardianship, treatment orders and the position of nearest relatives.)

It is only to be expected that, given the wide variety of patients able now to appear before MHRTs, there should be an equally large range of decisions to be made. Again, the list given here is not intended to be exhaustive merely to cover some of the major points to aid the discussions later. In general terms, for unrestricted patients, a tribunal may discharge a patient detained under the Mental Health Act but has a duty to do so if certain statutory criteria are met. If the patient was admitted for assessment, the tribunal shall order the patient's discharge if he is no longer suffering from mental disorder which warrants his detention in a hospital or his detention is no longer justified in the interests of his own health or safety or for the protection of others. If detained for treatment then roughly the same criteria apply. Also, for unrestricted patients, a tribunal can direct that a patient be discharged on a future date to allow aftercare arrangements to be made. Under the 1959 Act, patients had to be discharged immediately a MHRT had reached a decision and before aftercare had been arranged (Gostin, 1983). Now a tribunal can delay discharge, suggest a transfer to another hospital, reclassify the patients to another form of mental disorder or recommend transfer to guardianship.

For restricted patients, an MHRT must order an absolute or conditional discharge if the statutory criteria are fulfilled, in the latter case until the necessary arrangements have been made (Section 73(7)). Gostin points out that, as the Act now stands, a tribunal has no powers to recommend transfer or leave of absence. This, apparently was an unintended omission which is likely to be put right in the future. There is thus no possibility of granting a transfer for restricted patients in Special Hospitals who may need time in less restrictive surroundings. Yet this may be an important part of their gradual preparation for life in the community (Gostin, 1983, p. 44).

How and under what circumstances are cases referred to a tribunal? There are, roughly speaking, three ways. First the patient or nearest relative can make an application during the specified periods and according to Section 66 above. Second, the Home Secretary (for restricted patients) or the Secretary of State for Social Services can refer a case to a tribunal at any time. Finally, there is an automatic review, introduced by the 1983 Act to act as a safeguard against patients who did not take the opportunity to make an application perhaps because they lacked the ability or initiative or because they were unaware of their rights. Another important change accompanying the 1983 Act is that there is now legal aid and other forms of assistance for patients wanting to be represented before a tribunal. Legal representation has been made available for all applicants to a tribunal since 1 December 1982 under the Assistance by Way of Representation Scheme (ABWOR; see DHSS, Circular HN(83)37).

These then are the bare bones of the tribunal scheme. The 1983 Act has extended the scheme and the number of tribunals held is expected to increase greatly, probably by as much as five times compared to the situation under the 1959 Act. This is largely due to the new provisions and particularly for patients detained under Section 2, the 28 day order. It will be remembered that MHRTs are empowered to consider the need for continuing detention and, where it no longer exists to direct the patient's release. Unlike the Mental Health Act Commission, tribunals are not a forum for complaint although, I suppose, there is no reason why members should not refer matters to the commission if they considered practices to be sufficiently serious. There is a MHRT for each of the 14 National Health Service Regions for England and one for Wales. In this way all patients are covered.

There are other ways of securing discharge; the Home Secretary can order it, for a patient can petition for a writ of *habeas corpus*. I mention these for completeness' sake (see also Hoggett, 1984). I wish now to look at two features in greater detail: aftercare and MHRTs, beginning with questions of discharge generally.

Discharges generally

It will be remembered that a MHRT must discharge a patient if the patient is no longer suffering from mental disorder which warrants his detention in a hospital and his detention is no longer justified in the interests of his own health or for the protection of others. These conditions are relatively clear although, as will be shown later in this chapter, by no means easy to establish. For other patients, discharged through less formal channels, the question concerns the reasons for their discharge.

The conventional answer would be that they are no longer mentally disordered; they are cured or their symptoms are sufficiently relieved to allow them to take their places in the community. Where this is not so, their detention would doubtless be formally renewed if the patients were compulsory or the patients would remain in hospital if voluntary. The conventional or psychiatric answer hides matters which are a good deal more complicated. Social factors are I suggest as important as any in determining discharge. Patients who are disruptive are sometimes discharged early with notes on their files warning against future admissions. The number of these patients may be small but their presence points to a long-standing problem in mental hospitals which concerns the extent to which disruptive patients can be allowed to affect or jeopardise the recovery of others. I am not making a criticism of the practice of discharging such patients, merely pointing to the way in which decisions concerning discharge are rarely wholly psychiatric. Then, too, there are the home circumstances of patients: in the manner in which, for example, elderly patients are discharged it seems there are intricate social networks where the psychiatrist may be involved in bargaining with other departments (particularly social services departments) to provide the necessary social supports. Patients unable to secure such support tend to remain longer in hospital. Third, and finally, patients with heavy role expectations are more likely to be discharged early than those with correspondingly fewer. So for example a woman with (say) three children aged under five years living at home with husband or relatives is more likely to be discharged early than a similarly placed patient with no role expectations.

Then there are hospital policies, perhaps influenced by central government controls (fiscal or otherwise) to consider. The current trend towards 'community care' which involves what Scull (1983) refers to as the 'decarceration movement' is a deliberate attempt to close certain mental hospitals and discharge patients into the community. It is beyond the scope of this chapter to enter that debate, I wish only to bring into relief the general question of central government policies as they affect discharges and (for that matter) questions of admissions too.

There is also that abiding problem in psychiatry as to what constitutes patient recovery or cure. Cure in psychotherapy may be considered to have taken place when patient and psychoanalysts are in agreement. This is a little slick, perhaps, except that it points to the value systems of the psychiatrists as a determining factor. It points also to the paucity of objective measures of agreed criteria of improvement, the oft ill-defined aims of treatment and the heterogeneous nature of the disorders selected for treatment (Clare, 1983). In the latter, mental hospitals treat and cope with a wide range of patients, some neurotic able to benefit from the more gentle forms of psychotherapy others floridly psychotic. The psychiatrist dealing with the chronic patients might be prepared to settle for partial relief of the symptoms with some improvement in the behaviour and social functioning of the patient. If he did that of itself, it might be necessary to permit discharge although falling far short of a cure in the strict or accepted sense of the term.

I mention these points to raise doubts and questions about matters which are presented in the legislation as comparatively simple yet turn out, on closer inspection, to be complex. More often than not, decisions concerning patients' discharge involve an amalgam of factors (some psychiatric, some not) where the judgment of the psychiatrist has to be exercised. The discharge of patients must always be problematic. There is nothing certain about discharging patients any more than admitting them, and this applies as much to MHRTs as to individual psychiatrists. In the same way that diagnosis is considered an art rather than science, so too it seems is the decision about discharge.

Aftercare

In the 1983 Act, Section 117 imposes a duty to provide aftercare services for certain categories of mentally disordered patients who have ceased to be detained and have left hospital. It is not clear from the legislation if this will mean that patients will be forced to undertake aftercare. If so, I argue later in the chapter, this may be an unwelcome step. Nor is it entirely clear how aftercare provisions under Section 117 are or will be put into practice. At the time of writing (1985) only one local authority has allocated money for aftercare (MIND, 1985, personal communication). Otherwise nothing has changed. We are back again to the 'ideology of entitlement' argument given in Chapter 4, except that some lawyers are suggesting that this section of the Act, unlike those which recommend that local authorities provide services generally might be enforceable. Some lawyers say Section 117 deals with a well-defined group of patients and is specific in its intentions. Others, less optimistic, regard it as a persuasive tool which can be used to prise additional money from central government funds as and when necessary – i.e. compared to the National Health Services Act 1977 it is at least understandable. Most local authorities seem less than enthusiastic, believing that they will be involved in additional expenditure which they can ill afford during periods of financial restraint. Assume that lawyers and local authorities were enthusiastic about aftercare, what then? Is it to be welcomed? Many who gave evidence to the Butler Committee thought it was: they stressed the importance of helping with the patients' adjustment on discharge, of reducing the stigmatising effect of a compulsory order, or of helping with employment or accommodation etc. Some considered aftercare should be compulsory for a patient on a hospital order, others that supervision orders be added to all hospital orders. (HMSO, 1975, para. 8.2) The Butler Committee whilst retaining its enthusiasm for aftercare did not think it would be right to impose statutory requirements, especially with powers of recall, and did not think any further legal provision was justified. The government accepted this view although it had to concede over the general provisions of Section 117.

Before entering the details of the debate I wish to look at some general features of aftercare, and to make comparisons with the legal system. In the penal system aftercare can be either statutory or voluntary. In the former it lasts for a fixed period, the offender is allocated a supervisor (usually a probation officer or social worker) and there are powers of recall. Voluntary aftercare lacks formal requirements; there is usually no fixed allotted period and no corresponding powers of recall. Whether statutory or not, the aim is the same: to help the patient to readjust after a period of institutional life, to pick up the threads of his life again and to have assistance of a material or social kind. It is avowedly humanistic but a form of social control nonetheless. It operates as an auxiliary institution to the main institution. From research in the criminological field, aftercare appears to be operated by the responsible agencies according to one of two models: first the neutralisation model, which attempts to reduce the less attractive features of institutional life; second the continuation model, which attempts to build on the more attractive features (such as continuing with regular work habits etc). Sometimes the models merge, sometimes not. When they do it is possible that one offender may be subject to both models over the same (or different) periods of time, where the supervisor attempts to reduce, say, the patient's dependence on the institution and to encourage self reliance, yet at the same time to encourage the patient's interest in certain forms of work initiated by that institution. It is rare for patients to receive material help without being subject to one or both of these models: the tendency in modern social welfare is to do more than provide the basic necessities, there is nearly always an additional aim to influence behaviour, however slightly.

One can see that aftercare might be of value. At the humanistic level, statutory aftercare may help patients leaving institutions and, for these purposes, we are talking mainly of statutory forms. Patients may require periods of adjustment whether it be adjustment to family life, to work or to the countless other types of situations that make up daily lives. For the homeless, there may be problems relating to accommodation; for those whose mental disorder is in retreat but present nonetheless there are additional problems relating to personal relationships, the side-effects of medication, and the loss of security that institutional life can often bring. For the alcoholic (and although alcoholism is no longer a form of mental disorder warranting detention, some mental patients have problems with alcohol), outpatient-treatment facilities need to be arranged and encouragement granted at the appropriate time. At the control level, temporary lapses need to be corrected, sometimes with the threat of sanctions; work habits need to be instilled; an orderly regime must be created. For patients with a tendency to wander or have a restlessness which is self destructive, conditions of residence may need to be enforced. Guardianship, as presently constituted under the 1983 Act, is not satisfactory; the powers of the guardian are too narrow.

There are other ways in which statutory aftercare could help. Might it not be that hospitals would disharge patients earlier on the certain knowledge that they were being cared for in the community? Some think it might. Patients might be released on licence, similar to the method used in parole, although the parallel is slightly misleading because the parole licencee is still serving his prison sentence while on licence and cannot complain of being supervised and being liable to recall (HMSO, 1975, para. 8.3). Even so, the model of parole is a useful one, for the aim in parole is to reduce the length of time spent in prison by providing statutory supervision of discharge. If the licencee's behaviour is unsatisfactory, he can be recalled. The old borstal licence (now replaced by youth custody) operated on similar lines. Offenders were released when their training had reached a satisfactory level; while on release they were subject to a fixed period of licence. Of course, if statutory aftercare were to be introduced, it might be necessary to produce a type of licence different from that in the penal system whilst retaining the basic aims. Patients subject to a statutory after.care could still be eased into the community; if hospital authorities considered the services adequate, then discharge dates could be brought forward.

How would such aftercare provisions operate? We can ignore the restricted patients, for statutory aftercare exists for them. We are talking therefore of offender patients on hospital orders or the like and non-offender patients committed under civil commitment procedures. Consider first voluntary aftercare, for there are interesting lessons to be learned here from the field of criminology. In the first place, voluntary aftercare is rarely used to its full advantage. Most offenders are prepared to accept a limited form of material help but are less eager to accept assistance with forms of personal or self-adjustment. It is not difficult to see why: experiences in prison are unpleasant, and the offender is more often than not eager to forget them as quickly as possible. To accept voluntary aftercare is to be reminded of those experiences. Moreover, most offenders see the type of assistance offered as being patronising. They see their sentence as a debt to be paid and claim that they are quite capable of managing their own affairs on release. Paradoxically the type of work experience received in the prison, and the type of trade learned is the type of work they least wish to try on release. Again, one can see why: they would be reminded of the prison. Then there are the numbers of prisoners. The sheer volume makes it impossible to provide adequate aftercare facilities: in England and Wales about 100 000 prisoners are released each year. Moreover, the length of sentences is usually short, 6 months or less, making it extremely difficult to plan aftercare for every prisoner. About 10 000 additional probation officers would need to be appointed, with a similar number working inside the prison, if this system were adopted.

It may be unwise, even hazardous perhaps, to continue to draw parallels with the penal system; there are, however, sufficient common features to allow some inferences to be gleaned. Firstly, there is no groundswell of interest from mental patients to suggest they want extensive aftercare arrangements. Secondly, there are the problems of the numbers of patients to be dealt with, that is, numbers are roughly comparable with releases from prisons. Finally it is expected, and I put it no higher than this, that mental patients too may not wish to be reminded of their period in the mental hospital. Having been considered 'cured' they may wish to run their own lives without assistance from health authorities or whatever.

Statutory aftercare is an altogether different matter. It involves sanctions and recalls. If introduced, it would need a decision on the length of aftercare to be offered. There would also need to be a decision about the service deemed suitable to run it, about administrative costs and a commitment on behalf of the hospital to deal with patients who failed to abide by the statutory conditions: that is, if one could decide on the conditions to be inserted. These could be 'good behaviour' perhaps, or 'symptom-free', 'settled work habits' or even 'conditions of residence'. The conditions would need to be more pronounced and strident than those for guardianship for there would be no point otherwise in providing a duplicate service. When such a service is under way, might it not begin to look very much like aftercare in the penal system? Would this not put further strain on the civil commitment procedure if patients know that they had periods of statutory supervision on discharge? The answer is most probably yes.

What of the empirical evidence to support aftercare? The Butler Committee quoted with approval research by Nigel Walker and Sarah

McCabe. The Committee said 'Research has shown that there is some evidence that any form of contact by the hospital or social services with offender patients after their discharge from hospital is associated with a lower probability of reconviction and a more stable employment record and we have no doubt that it is highly desirable that they should receive after care' (HMSO, 1975, para. 8.3) Set against this, are the volumes of empirical work in the criminological field where at best (and at its most charitable) the conclusions are that the case for statutory or voluntary after care has not been proven. Statutory aftercare sometimes makes re-conviction rates worse. More often than not it has little or no effect. Sometimes it makes a marginal difference in reducing re-conviction rates over a short period, but these return to expected levels thereafter.

It may be undesirable to continue pointing to the penal system and making comparisons there, except that some patients are offenders, occasionally with criminal records prior to hospitalisation who may have been through the aftercare system already. Even if the parallels are not clear we should be unwise to ignore the evidence from the penal system before embarking upon a lengthy detailed or comprehensive system of aftercare. It is interesting too that identical arguments were once made for prisoners as are now being made for mental patients; that is, assistance was required to help prisoners re-adjust to the real world on release, that courts would be encouraged to give shorter sentences knowing that aftercare facilities existed and so on. Nothing of the sort happened, and those aims were not realised. Whilst we may know (or think we know) what ex-prisoners need, there is a small but enticing gap that cannot easily be bridged between knowing what people need and providing or meeting those needs. Where is the expertise which helps patients or prisoners to adjust? It is certainly not available in the penal system, or not available in abundance.

I am suggesting that we should be very wary indeed about moving in the direction of providing aftercare (particularly statutory aftercare) for mental patients, for that is the logical extension of Section 117. I am not saying mental patients are or will be free from problems on discharge but that we seem unable to provide the expertise to deal with these problems. It is not a good thing in itself to raise expectations that cannot be fulfilled. Statutory aftercare, with its additional emphasis on control, would I am certain be another control mechanism adding to the numerous ones already in existence. The evidence to support the case for aftercaré is meagre. For all its humanitarian overtones, and for all its claims to help patients on discharge, the reality may turn out to be quite different. It is a road down which I think we ought to be reluctant to travel and it is therefore wrong in my view to raise expectations that things could be otherwise. In saying this I am not denying the valuable assistance to some mental patients in the provision of halfway houses, hostels or whatever. There is a difference between this and providing blanket provisions for all mental patients and a world of difference between these and the hint of statutory aftercare implied in Section 117. Certainly let us provide extra provisions for discharged mental patients but keep these provisions voluntary, or even keep them as part of a homeleave scheme. Unless we know more of the intentions implied under Section 117 I think we should be very wary of what is being offered.

Mental Health Review Tribunals

Mental health review tribunals (MHRTs) are the most official and formal methods of discharge for detained patients. The patient's right to appeal to a MHRT provides certainty, protects his rights on matters of detention and discharge through a multidisciplinary approach. For this reason, MHRTs are not courts: the aim is less towards the adversarial model of justice normally practiced in Britain but towards the inquisitorial model. This has both advantages and disadvantages. The advantages are that the patient may feel less overawed than he would have done otherwise and tribunal members can probe into matters which an adversarial model tends to inhibit. On the other hand, the traditions of justice within Britain (and the assumptions bound up with those traditions) tend to be caught up with an adversarial view. It is difficult for MHRTs to marry different systems without losing something and weakening, both at the same time. How far it is possible to allow tribunal members a relatively free hand without offending canons of natural justice is difficult to assess.

The structure of the tribunal comprising as it does the legal, lay, and the medical members produces its own set of tensions. Fennell (1977) noted how tribunals tend to resemble a case conference where the medical member dominates by discussing the finer points of psychiatry with the hospital authorities. From my experience this form of medical dominance appears to be less pronounced where the chairman is a circuit judge or a person of similar standing. Even so, there is still the tension between the requirements of justice and the expertise of psychiatrists; they may even become incompatible.

Then there is the question of the patient's rights to see medical notes or to be aware of the nature of the psychiatric medical examination. Although the patient (in almost every case) has the right to see the medical report prepared by his doctor for the tribunal, neither he nor his representative has a right to see his medical notes although an independent doctor instructed by the patient can do so. The right to see medical notes is a problem that plagues so many areas of our life: medical psychiatric reports are not shown to defendants in the criminal courts although reports by probation officers and social workers are (for adult offenders at least). There is no right to see medical reports in civil cases such as adoption (nor does it appear there is a right to see other reports there either) or in other cases relating to child care. Why is this so? Apparently the grounds lie in the area of medical benevolence; that is, the physician may know something disturbing about the patient's medical condition about which it would be unwise (in the patient's best interests) to inform him. I can see no justification for this view.

A report, medical or otherwise, is about the patient who presumably trusts his physician although the trust apparently needs not be reciprocated. I am heartened therefore to see two recent resolutions which would grant the patient the right to see medical reports. The first from the American Hospital Association which, as far back as 1973, produced its Bill of Rights for patients. This document, which had no legal authority, was used as a model by several government bodies in North America which have produced legally binding Bills of Rights. Then in January 1984 the European Parliament formally tabled a resolution inviting the European Commission to submit as soon as possible a proposal for a European Charter on the Rights of Patients. Among the listed rights were 'the rights to information concerning diagnosis therapy and prognosis, the patient's rights of access to his own medical data . . .' (Faulder, 1985). How much better would it have been had the British government produced a similar initiative without having to wait again for that of the European Commission. (It is to be hoped too that when implemented there will be no clause which means that psychiatric patients will not be included particularly for patients appearing before a tribunal.)

It would have been better also had the British government taken the initiative itself over reforming tribunal procedures in the first place, rather than responding to the European Court. In the celebrated case of X v. United Kingdom, in a judgment given on 5 November 1981, the European Court of Human Rights held that under Article 5(4) of the European Convention, a detained patient has a right of access, at certain intervals to a judicial body to determine the justification for continued detention. Under the 1959 Act, a MHRT could only advise the Home Secretary, the Home Secretary could accept or reject that advice without giving reasons. The European Court held that a MHRT having an advisory power did not constitute a judicial body. Under the 1983 Act, tribunals have power to discharge patients subject to a restriction order – this change was instituted in order to abide by the European Court's earlier decision. Yet, strangely enough, the Home Secretary still retains power to discharge a patient absolutely, the tribunal's power running concurrently with the Home Secretary's. Will the Home Secretary discharge a patient who has not been seen by a tribunal? Almost certainly not, but the Home Secretary may still discharge a patient where the tribunal has decided not to.

The case of *X* v. United Kingdom is interesting in a number of respects. Firstly that it prompted the British government to do something about the then existing tribunal procedure and, as a result, it greatly strengthened MHRTs under the 1983 Act. The second is that *X* himself was a conditionally discharged patient from Broadmoor Special Hospital who was recalled by the Home Secretary acting on information from the patient's family and supervising officer. The European Court said that the Home Secretary must give reasons for his recall and that the patient had the right to a judicial hearing. What the European Court was saying amongst other things was that the burden of proof must rest with those who are doing the detaining and that they must also justify their actions. I see no reason to dispute this view for, under the earlier system, executive power was unbridled, producing insecurity for those likely to be subject to that power. Yet in spite of the changes under the 1983 Act, a residue of the older attitude remains. MHRTs seem to operate as if the burden of proof is on the patient to show why he should be discharged rather than on the hospital to show why the patient should continue to be detained. There is an implied suggestion that a patient should prove his sanity. It is difficult enough to show that one is no longer dangerous, given a previous offence or behavioural record, but at least there are some objective tests to go on (i.e. past and current behaviour). How can one prove that one is sane?

For all the advantages of the MHRT system, it fits uneasily in the general scheme of things. The composition of the tribunal (the legal, medical and lay member) is different from that which made the earlier decision on admission. There is no social worker on the MHRT – nor incidentally was there a legal member when the patient was admitted unless he came via the Court. Why is there not? Whatever the reason, MHRTs create the impression that it is considerably more important to get out of hospital than to get in. If the social worker and relative are central to the admission procedure then they ought also to be central to the discharge. If the lawyer is to protect legal rights, or ensure legality about matters of discharge then this should also be the case at admission. Of course, there may be logistical reasons why lawyers cannot be present when the patient is admitted but they do not apply to the social worker and relative who could attend tribunal hearings. The social worker could be present as a full tribunal member. It is a curious system which provides different standards and more rigour for matters of discharge than admission.

In saying this I am not criticising the MHRT and indeed welcome the attended opportunities granted to patients to have a Tribunal hearing. These provisions in the 1983 Act are worthy of support. Why should things be left there? Why not automatically include tribunal hearings for all cases, for patients whose treatment orders are being extended, or for long-stay informal patients who may languish in hospital without consideration of their predicament. More importantly, why not use the tribunal system as a means of granting an appeal against admission. I have said elsewhere that there is something very wrong with a system which does not grant a right of appeal for non-offender patients (Bean, 1980). Offender patients have such a right through the normal procedures of the criminal law, thereby adding to the paradox. The proposal I suggested (Bean, 1980) was to allow patients the right of appeal within 36 hours, the appeal to be before the magistrates' courts. If that proposal was unacceptable because it re-introduced the courts, then why not use the MHRT instead? It would not be impossible for lawyers to devise rules and procedures for such a hearing, nor for hearings to be arranged at such short notice. Without such a provision, the imbalance will continue.

Section III

Patients' rights

CHAPTER 8

Consent and treatment

It may seem a paradox, even a contradiction perhaps, to talk of consent and psychiatric treatment at one and the same time. If so then perhaps we need to recognise further the influence of earlier legislation which defined much of our thinking. The 1890 Lunacy Act for example, gave medical superintendents powers to administer treatments to certified patients without the patient's consent. These powers were simply transferred to the 1959 Act, according to the official interpretation at the time. Under the 1959 Act, or more specifically under Section 26 the treatment order, patients could be given all forms of treatment without their consent. At that time this was considered a normal and appropriate procedure, and indeed was so until quite recently.

Certainly the 1959 Act said nothing specifically about consent. But then, it wouldn't: consent was not part of the prevailing world view. The right to receive treatment was seen as more important, for treatment it was thought would enable patients to live more happy and useful lives. It is interesting therefore to see how consent was ignored. The Percy Commission justified compulsory detention according to the nature of mental disorders: that is patients may not know they are ill, and if they are unwilling to receive the form of care considered necessary there was a strong likelihood that unwillingness was due to a lack of appreciation of their condition, deriving from the mental disorder itself. By definition therefore, mental patients were unable to give consent – a neat tautological argument illustrating again the ease by which simple definitions can cast aside important policy questions. The climate has of course changed, not just in England and Wales but worldwide. Consent has become a contemporary issue, and the Percy Commission's arguments are no longer seen as acceptable.

The 1983 Act contains somewhat complicated procedures relating to consent. Indeed Part IV of the Act, and its attendant regulations (the Mental Health (Hospital, Guardianship and Consent to Treatment Regulations) 1983, No. 893) are, in my view, some of the most radical features of the Act – at least on the surface, although as will be shown later they do not go very far. Officially, consent to treatment was introduced into the 1983 Act by a wish on behalf of the government to remove existing uncertainties and to define the extent to which treatment for mental disorder can be imposed (DHSS, 1978 para. 6.14), but there was more to it than that. The desire to move away from the earlier form of paternalism, a sense of disillusionment with certain forms of psychiatric treatment, and the influence of some pressure groups such as MIND all helped push the government towards accepting consent, albeit in a limited form, as a worthy principle. It remains to be seen whether the Act has realised those aims.

It would be surprising if it did, and I say that without rancour or without wishing to belittle current legal achievements. The whole area is beset by uncertainties. It opens up questions earlier ignored, it produces professional rivalry and a variety of definitions. Consider, for example, professional rivalry. Kaufman *et al.* (1981) discovered fundamental differences in the manner in which psychiatrists and lawyers saw consent. Psychiatrists insisted they had a duty to make decisions on behalf of and in their patient's best interests whilst lawyers emphasised the patient's autonomy and self-interest. Psychiatrists assumed that diagnosis of mental disorder was sufficient justification for proceeding with almost any form of treatment, lawyers did not (Kaufman *et al.* 1981). Consider too the variety of definitions. Consent can be seen as the right to refuse all forms of treatment, or the right to refuse some but not others, or the right to refuse initially but to have that right taken away later or by a surrogate. There is real consent, informed consent, and (would you believe it?) future and limited consent. In order to pick our way through this, or as Gordon and Verdun-Jones (1983, p. 56) call it the Scylla and Charybdis of contemporary psychiatry [they note wryly the fate of an earlier mariner on that voyage], we can start by taking a broad overview before moving to the specifics of the 1983 Act.

Consent generally

Modern legal thinking on consent has been shaped and fashioned by the common law which respects the right of lay persons to decide what shall be done with their bodies. Children below a certain age cannot, however, give consent; furthermore, where a person has a notifiable disease or is carrying an organism capable of causing one, a Justice of the Peace (or sheriff in Scotland) can order the person to be medically examined and removed to a hospital and detained there. Generally speaking, any action which involves the use or the threat of force, however slight, upon the person will amount to a breach of the common law, unless there is consent or some specific legal justification for acting without it (Hoggett, 1984, p. 193).

In Britain the common law has protected the personal and bodily interests of the individual through the law of trespass. The administration of treatment to a person without his consent constitutes battery, apprehension without consent is an assault. The law of trespass, a tort, upholds the common law principle that a person should be able to refuse decisions about his wellbeing even if the proposed treatment is likely to benefit him. Consent may be given expressly or implied by conduct; in the latter, a man by putting out his arm to receive an injection implies consent (Gostin, 1983, p. 48). Consent may also be implied in matters of urgent necessity. In common law patients unable to give their consent because, say, they are unconscious, are presumed to have done so. They cannot then take action for trespass if it was known in advance that they had no objection to treatment. Such treatment may involve the use of lifesaving methods of the most extreme form. The question then arises to what extent can urgent necessity include, say, a sudden violent outburst by a patient in mental hospital? The Butler Committee thought it could. 'Certain eventualities such as the need to restrain a patient during a violent episode by the injection of a tranquiliser or to use medical procedures to save the life of a patient who lacks understanding would be covered by common law, treatment being justified on the grounds of presumed consent or necessity' (HMSO, 1975, para. 3.57). Some lawyers would disagree. Even so, and whatever the rights or wrongs of that argument there still exists considerable uncertainty concerning this and other areas of consent, some of which remains under the 1983 Act.

What then is meant by consent? That is, what do we mean when we say a person gives consent? To say X gives consent is to say X agrees to something that is happening to or is about to happen to him. It may be something that is given, or done to him and he accepts and agrees to that. Later he may not like the outcome and may regret having given consent, but this does not affect consent in the first instance. In order to give consent there must be some degree or amount of information given; X cannot be said to give consent to Y if he knows nothing of Y. There must also be a level of responsibility, for consent cannot be given by someone (e.g. a child) who is unable to make meaningful decisions. There must be an element of choice too, for X cannot be said to consent to Y if the agreement was extracted under coercion and agreed because he had no option. Consent implies free will or choice, it does not occur for those who believe in the general doctrine of determinism or where individuals are said to be behaving as automatons. Finally, consent must be related to something specific, for consent does not imply giving consent to everything; if it did, it would reduce the person as a human being, rendering him unable to make choices for himself.

Definitions of consent, including those described above, indicate a bias at the outset, and some would say a bias towards a certain type of political theory where rights relate to property rights and private ownership. I think that must be so, for consent implies ownership of a sort and ownership is a political concept. Any discussion of consent must proceed therefore on that basis. It contains a normative and political component which is bound up with a certain type of social order. Consent could not be welcomed for example by the out and out collectivist who might see it as a way of obstructing the social order. In contrast, consent has generally been welcomed by liberals who distrust all who have power and measure freedom by the strengths of those barriers which prevent intrusion into the individual's private world. I mention all this because it is as well to recognise the direction in which I shall be moving throughout this chapter. To assume, as I have, that consent is a good in itself and to assume too that part of its value is to enlarge freedom is to take on board a certain moral, social and political attitude.

Before entering the debate on consent as it applies to the 1983 Act, I would like first to examine some of the features of consent as defined above. It is not suggested that those given here are exhaustive, rather they constitute some of what we imply when we talk of consent. Nor is the order intended to imply priority, although awareness of self and surroundings must be regarded as central to any discussion. These features are: (i) awareness, which concerns the patient's condition and his ability to give consent; (ii) information and (iii) coercion, which concern the social millieu in which consent should, or should not operate; (iv) tidies up the definition by insisting that consent must apply specifically. The final section deals with matters where consent is unable to be given by the patient. This form of presentation differs from that adopted in the 1983 Act where the emphasis is on the types of treatment classified according to severity. That is the most severe treatments have the most restrictive procedures attached to them. I wish to approach the problem from the position of the patients believing that this is a more interesting exercise and likely to be the direction in which we in England and Wales shall move in the future.

Awareness

To say a person is aware of himself and his surroundings is to say more than that he has sensations but to show that actions follow on the basis of being able to evaluate his position. Sensations may be part of awareness, but awareness involves more; it involves evaluating sensations in moral terms. When we say a person is aware of himself we mean he is self-conscious and that, being conscious of self, he is also conscious of his surroundings. Consciousness of self includes beliefs, attitudes and thoughts, where it is necessary to know of existence and then to assess those thoughts in terms of origins, consistency or whatever. In this sense awareness, is a moral proposition involving varying levels of personal evaluation.

We can avoid the more detailed and lengthy debates on the nature of awareness by asserting in a matter of fact way that awareness implies making judgments about oneself. To give consent to something is part of that process. To be aware involves setting out the boundaries of one's life and dealing with others accordingly. It implies, although it cannot be taken for granted, that others – similarly aware – will also behave morally.

Yet, there are degrees of awareness; some people and at some times are more aware than others. Some, at one end of a continuum, remain aware of themselves at all times, others (at the other end) have never been nor will ever be. Instances or examples of this abound, among mentally impaired children or demented adults, to name but two groups. Some people may have periods of awareness punctuated by periods without it. What then? Again, and in a matter of fact way, those not aware ought not to be dealt with in a less moral way than those who are, for morality means respecting all persons whether aware or not. That some people lack this essential feature in the provision of consent is neither here or there in terms of the way they are dealt with generally, unless that is there are good grounds for saying that this should be so. Given the nature of their condition there may indeed be such grounds to justify providing different treatments being given. Some patients should perhaps be given greater care and respect, others given preferential treatment or additional assistance but none given less. Procedurally, distinctions need to be made between those who are aware and those who are not, and between those with varying degrees of awareness.

At the procedural level patients who have no knowledge of their position or of their current predicament lack the necessary degree of awareness to make decisions. Nor can they be aware if they do not know the moral quality of their acts, which may also include not knowing their thoughts, beliefs and attitudes. There is more to awareness than this. Mental patients, some of them anyway, are subject to rapid alterations in personality, mood swings or changes which indicate that they are 'not themselves'. Or to use F.H. Bradley's term, they are not self same. (Bradley, 1927, Chapter 1). That is, they have undergone some personality change, perhaps over a lengthy period so they are no longer recognisable. They behave in ways considered strange according to previous patterns of behaviour. They react differently from hitherto and may even produce and promote different reactions in others. At this time, patients who lack self sameness could also be seen as lacking awareness, for such changes suggest that previous ways of looking at the world (and views borne of earlier experiences) have been suspended, temporarily or otherwise. We would be right therefore to see those persons as being likely to make less sound judgments than hitherto.

This latter point implies that assessment of patients' awareness needs not be a professional exercise. Consider it this way: patients who are not self same may also have periods or phases when they are, for mental disorder is often punctuated by periods of lucidity. Assessments of the patient would be by those with prior knowledge of him, able to identify the necessary periods in which awareness occurs. Self sameness therefore has to be based on previous personal contact. This does not exclude a professional role which may involve current assessments of the patient's knowledge of his surroundings, perhaps even knowledge of the moral quality of his acts, but it does not grant a professional monopoly either. Assessments need not be dominated by nor undertaken solely by professionals and indeed in assessments of awareness they probably have less expertise than others. Assessments become a shared responsibility, a difficult and time-consuming task but not impossible given the appropriate goodwill.

Self sameness, especially when linked to knowledge of the moral quality of a person's acts, forces us to recognise the integrity of the patient and the patient's ability to make decisions, however wrong we or others might see them. There was the celebrated case of the woman, aged 60, who refused to grant consent for breast surgery because she thought it would damage her chances of being a famous actress, even though she had never acted before in her life. Her decision was upheld by the appeal court on the grounds that it was no business of the court, or anyone else for that matter, to say her judgment was faulty or ill conceived (Gostin, 1979, p. 139). Her refusal to give consent when to all intents and purposes she was 'self same' and the court's refusal to overrule her, is to be applauded.

Less closely related to the other points, self sameness allows us to avoid falling into any number of well-baited traps, and there are many of those. One is that causes of the disorder, or rather knowledge of the causes somehow takes away the patient's ability to be aware of his condition. The problem is that writers such as Freud and Marx (to name but two) spoke of psychological or environmental factors as if they were forces similar to mechanical pushes and pulls or unconscious mechanisms which impelled men to behave in certain ways making them prisoners of their past or catching them up helplessly in an unwinding historical pattern. Yet these 'causes' are irrelevant to the basic question of whether a person is aware of what he does. Causes do not compel; they merely provide plausible explanations for why a person acts in the way he does. This is true for pharmacological or organic causes as well as for environmental ones: to know that, say, a demented person had the dementia caused by an organic condition has little to do with whether he or she is aware or responsible. It may explain the condition but questions of awareness have to be decided on the basis of other considerations.

Awareness itself however is of little value without other features being present, such as the information upon which to base ones decisions, on being free from coercion etc. Whilst it may be convenient to separate the various factors involved in consent, in reality they are closely interwoven. All rely on a moral commitment on behalf of the professionals and others to enable genuine consent to take place.

Information

It was said earlier that consent implies being given information, for X cannot be said to consent to Y if he knows nothing of Y. That much is obvious. What is less so is the amount of information to be given, and the manner in which it is to be delivered.

Take first the information to be given. Another of those well-baited traps suggests consent cannot and ought not to apply where the information is itself limited, or as in psychiatric treatment where there are too many unknown variables. For example how or why electroconvulsive therapy (ECT) works remains largely a mystery as do many other forms of psychiatric treatments. It follows then, or so the argument goes, that patients cannot be expected to give consent with such insufficient information. The argument is I think flawed for the amount of available information has nothing to do with consent. In Murphy's (1979, p. 418) terms 'Consent does not become uninformed in any relevant sense because there is a shortage of information'. Information is important so far as the patient is told what is known and also of what is not known and allowed to make a decision accordingly.

Related to this is another such trap: that the information itself is often highly technical and cannot be reduced or imparted without distorting it, thereby losing the content. So medical practitioners' understanding of mental disorders and the technical treatment involved will always be greater than that of a patient. Try as he will, a psychiatrist can never impart more than a fragment of the total relevant information, yet to do less is to mislead. For example knowledge of many treatments requires a detailed and lengthy study, the conclusions of which cannot be reduced to a simple statement of facts presented and digested by the untrained. Again, there is something in this of course. Technical jargon is often a shorthand way of reducing complexities to manageable terminology, and technicalities can become absurdities when reduced to simple language. The molecular structure of certain neuroleptics requires more than a short description of their content and effects in order to appreciate their subtleties and complexities. Yet whilst it may be difficult, time-consuming, even well nigh impossible to convey the full impact of the information, consent is about a moral commitment on behalf of the informer to provide information upon which the decision can be made. In the same way that consent of a sort can be obtained from say a mentally impaired person who may agree to anything, so consent of a sort can be obtained by bludgeoning people with technical information. That is not however what is meant by consent.

Information of itself is the bare bones as it were, the skeleton which requires something more to make it lifelike. That comes from the way the information is given. To quote Murphy (1979, p. 423) again 'it is necessary to create an environment which makes it likely that the right questions will be asked by the patient and those questions will be answered in a useful way – i.e. an environment which is conducive to calm reflective comfortable discussions and deliberation'. To say, as do some medical practitioners, that they have neither the time or the facilities is an objection to the means rather than to the principle. The principle is aimed at assisting the patient to come to a considered decision, not about protecting the medical practitioner. Moreover, as a general rule, it would seem that the amount of information to be given must be related to or commensurate with the risk involved. Whilst it may not be necessary to spend a great deal of time discussing the effects of minor tranquillisers, carrying little risk it is (or should be) quite different for the major ones, or indeed for any treatment carrying a certain risk. It is therefore very important that the correct environment be provided, so that patients can deliberate and make the necessary decisions.

Aside from these procedural questions, issues of substance remain tantalisingly difficult. Some people require considerable amounts of information, some less; some people prefer to have no information at all. Some may get bewildered at the prospect of being given any amount of information whatsoever, some may ask but do not want the reply. Procedures and principles must, in the last resort, be put into practice and be dependent on a commitment and a judgment about what is acceptable. It is perhaps for reasons akin to this that in some countries there is 'informed consent' although, in the strictest sense of the term, consent always implies being informed. Presumably the aim is to add emphasis and, in doing so, to prevent manipulation by physicians or protect patients against well-meaning but ignorant ones (Murphy, 1979, p. 422). 'Informed consent' places the responsibility on physicians to provide relevant and up-to-date information. In England and Wales, valid consent is defined by the DHSS (1978, para. 6.23) as 'the ability given an explanation in simple terms to understand the nature, purpose and effect of the proposed treatments'. It is not clear how or why 'valid consent' differs from just plain ordinary consent for, by definition, consent must be valid (as it should be informed). Presumably this too was intended, to provide emphasis.

In spite of the various arguments in favour of consent (informed or otherwise) and the amount of information to be given, there remain numerous critics and sceptics. Some have argued that informed consent places too great an emphasis on what the patient gets or understands compared to what he wants (Goldstein, 1975, quoted in Hoggett, 1984). Others are even more dismissive, seeing consent as a myth or slogan believing that no one can be informed, or fully informed or even partially informed to make a decision, especially when it involves matters as technical and complex as psychiatric treatments. They would see valid consent as an equally empty term, for few (except the interested, intelligent and exceptionally alert) can understand the 'nature, purpose and effect' of any proposed treatment, unless that is they have had previous experiences and knowledge of those treatments. There will always, of course, be sceptics; yet, before one dismisses their scepticism as unworthy, it is as well to remember that their scepticism extends to all areas of medicine, not just psychiatry (Faulder, 1985). The problem with psychiatry is that the mental condition of the patient adds to the list of complications. That, if anything, should encourage us to redouble our efforts to provide adequate consent procedures for psychiatric patients, rather than surrender to those who may be scornful of such attempts.

Control and coercion

Control is an essential feature of mental hospital life. Control is exercised by the medical profession, assisted by paramedical and other professional personnel. This point is not weakened by emphasising other considerations,

such as the provision of psychiatric care to mentally disordered people
involving diagnostic, therapeutic and rehabilitative processes. Too often
the literature on psychiatry ignores or side-steps the control questions,
preferring to emphasise more morally appealing features such as the
availability of therapeutic facilities etc. When a compulsory order is made
the patient is being controlled (as he also is when violent or disruptive).
Similarly, when he is refused permission to leave hospital, or in countless other ways when dealt with by hospital staff. The informal patient
fares little better in the daily regimen except that controls at certain key
points are absent (one sociologist talks of the pinpricks of social control that
affect patients lives).

Consent to treatment (whatever form it takes) is a way of reducing
control, usually over formal patients and in one specific area of their lives.
The patient can exercise choice and obtain freedom where he could not
hitherto. However other forms of control are not necessarily affected; he
cannot leave the hospital, cannot exercise choices over the nature of the
hospital regime or make other decisions which were denied him earlier.
Certainly the right to consent provides an important freedom, the more so
when treatments are irreversible and dangerous, but it remains one freedom
nonetheless to be set against the loss of numerous others as a detained
patient.

If that freedom is to be exercised it must not involve coercion or fraud or
deceit. In an obvious sense there can be no consent if coercion is used: X
cannot be said to be consenting if agreement is extracted with the assistance
of Y's gun, or the patient is deceived into thinking he is doing something
else. Coercion neutralises consent. The problem with coercion, as it affects
mental patients (and for these purposes we shall ignore questions relating to
fraud or deceit), is that it is never as naked as that but may involve more
subtle threats of punishments, loss of privileges, threats of further detention
etc. Where psychiatric staff say 'we shall do this or that to you unless you
consent to this treatment' they are involved in coercion. Similarly when they
say 'we shall keep you in hospital unless you consent to this treatment' they
are also involved in coercion. (I am not saying this happens or happens
regularly, merely using this as illustrative of a point.)

Assume that hospital staff said to a patient 'unless you consent to this
treatment your condition will deteriorate'. Is coercion being exercised then?
It is not, according to the interpretation of coercion given here. For the
essential difference from coercion, as illustrated in these examples, is that
coercion takes unfair advantage of the patients vulnerability. The latter
does not. It accepts his position, provides him with a choice even though the

range of choices are limited (in this case, improvement as against deterioration). The same point was well made by Murphy when he said the core of the concept of coercion is moral not psychological. It is not about avoiding psychological pressure, for no greater psychological pressure could exist than in the latter example, but avoiding psychological pressure that is unfair. 'Coercion of a subject involves taking an unfair advantage of his vulnerability by proposing, unless he accepts a certain offer to treat him in a way that is unfair and in a way he has no power to resist' (Murphy, 1979, pp. 424–5). So, where consent is extracted with threats of punishment, loss of privileges and threats of further detention this is coercion for it takes unfair advantage of the patient's vulnerability. There is no coercion where the patient is placed under pressure, however severe, even though that pressure may involve life or death choices. A person is not coerced because he is pressurised; he is coerced when his vulnerability is exploited.

It could of course be argued that being put in the position of being a mental patient is by its very nature coercive; that is, the patient is vulnerable from start to finish for the regimen itself produces stress and hidden threats which involve coercion. This extreme view is contained in a judgment Kaimowitz v. Michigan (in Gostin, 1979, p. 151).

It is impossible for an involuntary detained patient to be free of ulterior forms of restraint or coercion when his very release from the institution may depend upon his cooperation with the institutional authorities and giving consent to experimental surgery. . . .

Involuntary confined mental patients live in an inherently coercive institutional environment. Indirect and subtle psychological coercion has profound effects upon the patients population. . . .

They are not able to voluntarily give informed consent because of the inherent inequality of their position. (July 10, 1973).

Such an extreme view must be set against the common law duty of care owed by hospital staff towards their patients. Hospitals have a duty to take reasonable care of their patients and this involves offering them the care and treatment which they need (Hoggett, 1984, p. 197). It is no doubt easy to find in England and Wales supporters for each view; the numerous inquiries on the conduct of staff in certain hospitals including the special hospitals are testimony to one, and the gratitude of certain patients testimony to the other. Neither should be dismissed, for both exist in the overall pattern of things and events.

Even if it were found that coercion existed throughout mental hospitals in England and Wales that is no reason to dispense with consent procedures. Rather, we should do all we can to remove coercion in all its forms. Coercion can be defined as social control unfairly wielded yet, by its nature, subtle and difficult to remove. It may come in the form of a promise to provide an early discharge or through some such similar approach. In prisons, inmates may be coerced into taking part in drug experiments as a condition of the award of parole. Where this is so, it operates for the benefit of those in power and authority to the unfair advantage of the inmates. As such, it cannot be justified. Control however is a different matter. It too requires justification as do all restrictions on freedom. It differs from coercion, however, in the manner in which it holds neither threats nor unfair promises.

Consent related to specifics

Very briefly, and for completeness sake, when we talk of consent we mean giving consent to a specific action or related actions – or at least we ought to, for we do not usually talk of consent which permits anything or everything done to us. That would imply a loss of respect for individuals as responsible human beings. Consent to a medical procedure would include authorisation to do what is normally done in respect of that procedure. Consent to ECT, for example, would provide authorisation for an anaesthetic or muscle relaxant – a reasonable course of such treatment, in accordance with accepted medical practice. Consent is given on the assumption that treatment will benefit the patient and not in the interests of science or medicine generally (Gostin, 1979).

Problems arise when consent is given to one type of treatment but during this course of treatment (often during an operation) a more serious situation is discovered. What happens then? If the newly discovered situation is classified as an emergency, the physician will be covered by the common law as it affects emergencies. If not, the physician should not proceed. (The common law is unclear on this, however; such action might be justified if the treatment was necessary for health if not for life.) The Canadian position is more satisfactory, distinguishing procedures which are necessary, that is unable to be postponed from those which are merely convenient. The former may be performed where the patient is unable temporarily to give consent, the latter may not (Gostin, 1979, pp. 141–2). It is not known how often such additional treatments are given in England and Wales, probably very often indeed. Where this is so, the physician proceeds on the basis of what is called future consent; that is he assumes the patient will be grateful and ratify the physicians decision later. Yet the physician should perhaps heed Lord Devlin's remarks when he said 'the common law does not consider an act done without the person's consent but for his benefit as deserving of reward . . . . The Good Samaritan is a character unesteemed by the English law' (quoted in Gostin, 1979, p. 133).

These four features, awareness, information, coercion and specificity involve most of what I take to mean when we talk of consent. They are not features easily reduced to simple statements nor do they raise questions which are likely to be readily solved. They have a timeless quality about them and will, I think, forever remain at the centre of the debate.

Consent and surrogacy

There remains the difficult and troubling issue of consent as it implies to children, and to others who are permanently and irredeemably unable to give consent. This is sometimes referred to as surrogate consent so that, when a person is judged to be incompetent, his consent cannot be granted or given. A surrogate is used to grant consent on that person's behalf.

Dealing first with children: as matters stand, children below a certain age have fewer rights than adults, and are often held less accountable. Parents and school teachers have duties to provide the child with care and support; parents have a duty not to neglect the child, not to expose him to moral danger or to allow him to be beyond control. Children normally cannot undertake contractual obligations and are not morally entitled to their own earnings, nor can they manage their own property. Moreover children younger than certain statutory limits are not allowed to vote, hold public office, work in various occupations, drive a car, buy alcohol or be sold certain kinds of reading material, quite apart from what they or their parents may wish. (Bean, 1980, p. 110). The age at which children assume various responsibilities and obligations varies. In England and Wales the prosecutable age is 10; they cease to be beyond control at 17; they can vote at 18, and so on.

In England and Wales children cannot legally give consent to medical treatment under the age of 16, but (as always) matters are never as clear cut as that. For example, there is a common law right of a minor below the age of 16 to consent on his own behalf (see Gostin, 1979) although the 1969 Family Law Reform Act seems to suggest otherwise. That 1969 Act also says that a minor can give consent over the age 16, yet it remains unclear as to what is the parent's position if the minor, aged between 16 and majority, through mental handicap or whatever, is unable or incapable of understanding the nature of consent.

An equally pressing problem arises when parents, acting on behalf of children give or do not give consent in matters in which others would take exception. The most obvious examples are where parents wish a young girl to be sterilised or refuse permission for the child to have a necessary blood transfusion. The usual solution is for the child to be made a ward of court and for the court to direct accordingly. Technically all children are wards of court, the making of a wardship order is only a recognition of a process and a means of formalising it (Spicer, 1984). Wardship has the important function of granting the State the right to intervene in matters between parents and child to provide protection when it sees parents failing to do so. In England and Wales there are then two authorities capable of acting on the child's behalf: the parents and the State where the latter has ultimate authority. I cannot and do not see how that ought to be otherwise; otherwise the situation would become dangerously close to one where children are the sole property of their parents.

Where the state intervenes under a wardship order it is likely to make decisions based on a conservative ideology. The courts rarely innovate nor are they often in the vanguard of new thinking. Occasionally that may be regretted. Yet in those relatively few instances where a wardship court becomes officially involved it is perhaps wisest to play safe rather than to be innovative. The court is guided by the doctrine of the 'best interests of the child' yet this is capable of wide intepretation, and its history over the last century has not always been one where the child's best interests seemed to have dominated. Regrettably it can and has been used to justify unpleasant forms of intervention in childrens' lives. Playing safe seems more commendable.

For adults unable to give consent because of extensive or complete psychosis there is the Court of Protection to manage their affairs if they are incapable of doing so. This Court of Protection applies only to matters of property and not to consent. There is also guardianship but, under the 1983 Act, the guardian has fewer powers than before. Under the 1959 Act the guardian had powers over the patient as if the patient were a 14 year old child (see Chapter 4). That no longer applies, although the 1983 Act may grant a form of consent to the guardian where the patient is living under a condition of residence. That is where a person under guardianship has to reside in accommodation and the patient must abide by the rules of that accommodation. It could be seen then that a condition of residence grants those enforcing the residence certain powers reaching over and above that of the guardian himself.

Clearly those unable to give consent require surrogates to act on their behalf. Who should those surrogates be? Those with similar values to the patient? Should the surrogate reflect the patients supposed wishes? If so, then must the surrogate be someone who knew the patient prior to the mental demise? What should be the duties of surrogates? Should they act in a wardship capacity reflecting more general social attitudes and making decisions on matters of public policy, or perhaps in some other way? All such questions can be highlighted again in that age-old question of Jehovah's Witnesses and blood transfusions. Suppose, for example, a person who is a Jehovah's Witness later becomes clinically demented and incidentally requires a blood transfusion. Should a surrogate be appointed from that sect or from another group (an atheist perhaps who regards those religious beliefs as simply odd; see also Murphy, 1979). We appear not to have given these questions much thought in England and Wales, yet they will I am sure become increasingly important.

Consent defined under the 1983 Act

Part IV of the 1983 Act, which includes Sections 56–64 is entitled 'Consent to treatment'. These nine sections break new ground in mental health legislation in England and Wales. In doing so, the law enters an area which is uncertain and where principles, procedures and the like become interwoven. Sometimes procedures turn out to be principles, sometimes not, and sometimes principles are more like procedures. We are back to the Scylla and Charybdis problem noted earlier. Whatever and however many criticisms there are, I think we should see the 1983 Act as a preliminary sally into an area where amendments will be made, and refinements will occur to adjust to those criticisms. It is doubtful if any government in the near future will remove consent from the statute book. The mood is otherwise and consent is here to stay.

It is important therefore to see consent in mental health as part of a wider set of arguments in medicine generally, and consent in all areas of medicine is apparently not immune from criticism (see Faulder, 1985). There the attack is not so much on matters of procedure in the formal sense, for hospital patients are presented with a consent form prior to treatment. Criticisms relate to the manner in which consent is interpreted and occasionally circumvented, and of the doctor–patient relationship which is one-sided and raises again the spectre of professional dominance. Faulder points to a long line of dissatisfactions with mainstream medicine; the title of her book '*Whose Body Is It?*' conveys the essential message.

Briefly, as far as the legal provisions in the 1983 Act are concerned, Section 56 sets out where consent shall apply, or rather shall not apply. It shall not apply to emergency patients, patients subject to guardianship or detained under Section 136 (see Chapter 4). It shall not apply to informal patients, with the exception of patients likely to receive certain types of irreversible treatments; the latter point justified by the Minister of Health on the basis that 'if a course of treatment is so drastic that a detained patients consent alone should not justify it . . . it is difficult to see why the same provision should not apply to an informal patient' (Parliamentary Debates, 1982, vol. 29. col. 1). In those situations where consent does not apply, the patient is in the same position as a non-psychiatric patient who can only be treated without his consent in certain emergency situations (Jones, 1983).

Section 57 is one of the most interesting and important sections. This section requires consent to be obtained from the patient and second opinions from others where treatments involve 'any surgical operations for destroying brain tissue or for destroying the function of brain tissue' (see 57(a)) and 'such other forms of treatments as may be specified for the purpose of the section by regulations made by the secretary of state' (Section 57(b)). The use of a second opinion is interesting in two further respects: first and most obvious, consent is required from the patient which presumably means taking into consideration most if not all of the points made earlier in this chapter. Second, parliament has decreed that consent given to the registered medical practitioner in charge of the patient is not sufficient warrant for such treatment to proceed. This section requires (under sub-section 2) that a patient shall not be given any form of treatment to which this section applies unless he has consented and a medical practitioner and two lay people appointed by the Mental Health Act Commission have certified that the patient has given real consent. Additionally, the Commission doctor has to certify having consulted two persons professionally concerned with the patient's care; one must be a nurse 'the other shall be neither a nurse nor a registered practitioner' – usually therefore a social worker, psychologist or someone of similar standing that the treatment should be given. Consultation must involve an exchange of information – although how much and of what nature is not specified. However, to add to the safeguards, Section 60 allows a patient to withdraw consent at any time whereupon treatment shall cease forthwith.

The type of treatment covered by this section involves psychosurgery, hormone treatments etc. ECT was included originally during the committee stage of the bill but subsequently withdrawn; it comes up under a later section of the Act (Section 58). To put the matter of psychosurgery in some perspective: in England and Wales, from 1979 to 1982, there were 207 psychosurgical operations on informal patients and 4 on detained patients (Special Standing Committee, 22nd Sitting, 29 June 1982, col. 832). These figures are consistent with a report by a psychiatrist in charge of the Geoffrey Knight psychosurgical unit in London, which reports one operation per week (or about 1000 operations carried out over the past 20 years). This unit was responsible for all but three of the psychosurgical operations in England and Wales in 1982 (Bridges, 1984).

During its passage through Parliament, two forms of criticism were directed at Section 57. The first relates to the requirement that the registered medical practitioner shall consult people who are outside the main ambit of the medical profession (i.e. social workers, psychologists). A letter from the National Schizophrenia fellowship to the Special Standing Committee says 'We would be quite happy if consultation with other professions was recommended but most certainly not to have this . . . quite ridiculous requirement'. A letter from Dr Hamilton and Dr Unwin of Broadmoor hospital stated 'we are firmly against any proposal that the independent psychiatrist should be required to consult any other professional person than a registered nurse concerned with the patients treatment' (col. 812). To repeat the point: 'consultation' in this respect includes the exchange of information and the giving and the seeking of advice (Jones, 1983).

The second criticism was concerned with the manner in which, under Section 57, psychiatric clinical decisions were to be subject to veto. Certain medical practitioners saw this as explicit criticism of their clinical work. It suggested to them that the psychiatrists' experiences appeared to render them untrustworthy to assess patients and to provide independent treatments. Bridges (1984), in charge of that psychosurgical unit mentioned earlier, went further predicting dire consequences: 'This country now seems to be adopting that essential American folly, long recognised by psychiatrists on this side of the Atlantic but so appealing to militant moralists the control of medical practice by means of statute law and committees with non-medical and non-professional members where doctors are in a minority'. Moreover consent 'is the thin end of an ominous wedge and those in other medical specialisms should watch developments closely'.

This is a predictable reaction from members of the British medical profession when their dominance is threatened. To talk of 'militant moralists' adds nothing to the quality of the debate and detracts from the main questions. These concern: the extent to which consultations with members outside the medical profession might be expected to produce a better patient service; how much information should be given on the patient's medical condition to those who have not been connected with the patients treatment hitherto; what should happen to psychiatrists if they refuse to consult; or, when consultation takes place, what should happen if the person consulted is by all accounts unreasonable and appears intent on obstruction rather than on cooperation. It would have been better to concentrate on these questions rather than trying to appear as if the World were still flat and Parliament deeply unreasonable. On the other point, that consultation is 'the thin end of an ominous wedge' and that 'other medical specialisms should watch developments closely' the answer is quite so. Psychiatrists have only themselves to blame. Regulations and control was imposed on them because they have not policed themselves, or changed with the spirit of the times. They clung to an outdated vision of psychiatry provided by the 1959 Act. Psychiatry has paradoxically become a public affair because the professionals seemed intent on keeping it private. The more it is kept private, the more it will become public.

To return to the more prosaic features of consent within the 1983 Act. Section 58 is concerned with treatment which requires consent or a second opinion. It should also be looked at in terms of Section 60. These sections are however difficult to understand. The legal drafting is sometimes obscure, permitting numerous interpretations. As I understand it, this section requires first that ECT cannot be given without consent – or rather statutory instruments relating to sub-section (a) specify that ECT cannot be given without consent, and if consent is not granted a second opinion is required.

Sub-section (b) requires that the administration of medicine shall not be given after 3 months unless the patient consents, or an independent medical practitioner has certified that the patient is incapable of giving his consent, or that the patient should receive treatment even though he has not consented to it. If the patient consents to the treatment, the responsible medical officer or an independent medical practitioner must certify that consent has been properly given.

There are numerous legal tangles relating to this sub-section and many claims that the legislation is doing more than it really is. As I see it, all it does is permit the patient to exercise consent after 3 months of treatment, or on day 1 if the treatment is ECT. Thereafter a second opinion is required if consent is not given. However it is not clear from the legislation what then happens if, after 3 months, the patient says he never consented to any of the treatments given but the physician said he did, or that he consented to some but not to others. I suggest a pragmatic solution: that is to begin with an assumption that consent had not been given at any time during the 3 months period and to provide a second opinion immediately after. Nor is it clear in the case of ECT when a second opinion should be required and what happens if the second opinion then authorises further ECT. Are there limits to the numbers of ECTs to be given?

Why select a 3 month period? Clearly, it was a compromise: in the parliamentary debates (Special Standing Committee, 29 June, col. 825) it was proposed that 1 month be sufficient but this was rejected; 'One month is too short. Within that period the registered medical officer has to assess the patient, relieve the initial symptoms, reach a diagnosis and plan the best possible treatment in consultation with other professionals and relatives' (col. 833). Three months was preferred: '. . . three months gives time for the psychiatrist to consider a treatment programme which suits the patient . . . It is long enough to allow a proper valuation and assessment . . . it is short enough to ensure the patients consent or a second opinion is obtained before a long term course of drug treatment gets too far ahead' (col. 833). This is not really true; 3 months is also long enough for a patient to have received too much of the treatment and to be unable to give consent, or to make a reasoned judgment as a result. It is interesting to note however that from October 1984 to 30 June 1985 a second opinion was required on 4032 patients who received medication of which 2146 (58%) received ECT (MIND: personal communication, 1985). So it appears that second opinions are being sought extensively.

Finally on these legal matters, Section 62 deals with urgent treatment, and states where Sections 57 and 59 shall not apply. Treatment can be given to the patient without his consent, if any of the following conditions apply. That treatment is considered necessary to save the patient's life or second, not being irreversible is immediately necessary to prevent a serious deterioration of his condition or third, not being irreversible or hazardous is necessary to alleviate serious suffering or finally, not being irreversible or hazardous is immediately necessary and represents the minimum interference necessary to prevent the patient behaving violently or being a danger to himself or to others. Sub-section 3 defines irreversible as having unfavorable, irreversible physical or psychological consequences, and hazardous if it entails significant physical hazard. So, for example, treatments which are irreversible but favourable would according to the Under Secretary of State include removal of a brain tumour and removal of a diseased thyroid (Special Standing Committee, 29 June 1982, col. 782). When such conditions exist, the need for consent is suspended.

An assessment of the law relating to consent

It is not easy to assess consent in relation to the 1983 Act except to say that the Act is at best a move in the right direction. At worst it can be seen as a limited exercise with chances lost and opportunities missed. Perhaps it is appropriate to say what the law does not do and begin from there. First it does not deal with informal patients who make up the bulk of the current admissions to mental hospitals – about 90%. Informal patients can presumably decide whether to accept or reject treatment. If they reject, then psychiatrists are faced with alternatives: to discharge them or place them on a compulsory order, in which case matters of consent then apply. It is not, however, as simple as this. In mental hospitals there are large numbers of informal patients, whether they be mentally impaired or demented, who may not have been admitted on a formal order whose detention is equally real. Being unaware of their surroundings only makes the order unnecessary, it does not alter their predicament. Lacking the physical and intellectual wherewithal to change their status or situation, a formal order exists for them as surely as it does for the compulsory patients. Informal patients are not covered by most of the consent procedures yet it seems they ought. The logistics of it would then become difficult, for the number of second opinions required would be prohibitive. In the same way that the criminal courts function well because 90% of those appearing before them plead guilty, so consent procedures work because a similar percentage are not involved in these procedures.

Second, consent procedures under the 1983 Act do not give rights which allow detained patients to refuse treatment, except in exceptional cases under the section relating to irreversible and dangerous treatments. The bulk of the procedures come under the so called 3 months rule where refusal to give consent can be overruled. The situation is the same with ECT. Refusal to consent may only delay matters in order that a second opinion may be called. In this sense, consent becomes a stalling tactic rather than an absolute right to refuse. In some instances, the right to give consent is dependent on the medical practitioner seeking a second opinion. Under Section 58 the registered medical practitioner must say that the patient has not consented to treatment and, in the medical practitioner's opinion, the patient requires that form of treatment. Only then will a second opinion be sought. The honesty and integrity of the medical practitioner is required and by the nature of things, no one will know when that is found wanting.

What then does the act do? Perhaps its greatest achievement has been to provide formally a set of procedures whereby consent can take place in conditions favourable to the patient and in an atmosphere where no such tradition had existed. This is no small achievement from which further improvements can grow. I think the 1983 Act should not be seen as being the last word on the subject. I would expect changes to be made in procedures: e.g. in an increase in the types of treatments warranting consent, and perhaps also changes in the 3 months rule. There may be developments in surrogate consent to bring into line those patients classified as informal whose conditions render them vulnerable, i.e. the demented elderly.

Then there are important secondary effects. The major one is that the legislation is likely to force psychiatrists to treat patients according to a central orthodoxy, thereby reducing maverick treatments and idiosyncratic methods. So, where patients refuse consent and a second opinion is required, the second opinion doctor is likely to suggest alternatives more in touch with conventional thinking. Excessive use of ECT is likely to diminish for the same reason, for the second doctor may be wary of authorising further lengthy treatments. So too with polypharmacy, and perhaps the excessive use of some of the major tranquillisers. There might also be other gains whereby patients believe themselves to be real people as opposed to objects or aggregates of symptoms and believe they are actively involved in their treatment. Who knows? Perhaps Faulder's hopes may be realised: medical practitioners may learn to talk to (rather than talk at) their patients, thereby helping to reduce some of the features that characterise the ugly class divisions of our society (Faulder, 1985).

This is for the future, and changes of that order require changes in the social structure which modern high technology medicine is unlikely to make without adequate directions. The 1983 Act was a start but there is much further to go. Consent procedures have not I fear shifted the relative power of medical practitioners in terms of their patients where the one is seen as knowledgeable, responsible and rational and other is not. The onus is still on the patient to show he is rational or aware unless proven otherwise. Things need not be like this. The opposite position is equally tenable namely that mentally disordered patients are aware and responsible and should be seen as such, unless proven otherwise. In asserting this I of course betray a belief in the plurality of values and in old-fashioned liberalism.

Yet I think there are good reasons for adopting this second presumption, for it views human beings as ends in themselves rather than objects needing treatment in order to be made into human beings. The presumption also avoids slipping into interpretations which are unwarranted, or rather accept that some patients behave in ways which seem entirely reasonable to them according to the life situation in which they find themselves. Furthermore, it forces consideration of the nature of awareness and makes awareness a focus of debate (i.e. what does awareness mean and how can it be determined?). Finally, it assumes that people are rational unless proven otherwise, placing the onus on those who dispute rationality to justify their position. Unhappily the trend in psychiatry has been away from this presumption, and for that we must thank or berate the pathology model so prevalent over the last 40 years or so. It has provided a model that assumes pathology amongst various client groups: that prospective adoptive parents are unsuitable unless proven otherwise, that delinquents are maladjusted unless proven otherwise, that unemployed are feckless unless proven otherwise, and so on. If nothing else, the question of consent has forced a reappraisal of that view.

Finally, it is important to recognise the method adopted for consent procedures under the 1983 Act. As I said at the beginning, consent is related to a supposed scale of severity of treatment so that those treatments being more severe (psychosurgery for example) require more elaborate procedures. Of course, these procedures apply only to detained patients. It was probably correct to begin this way, for it implies disapproval of certain treatments and presumably allows other treatments to be graded or regraded accordingly. It does not however concentrate on the patients themselves or to attempt to classify them in terms of their levels of awareness, or to begin to regulate the manner in which they receive information, or are free from coercion etc. I suggest the next step is to begin to move in that direction. In this chapter I have concentrated more on that latter view, believing it to be a means of redressing the balance.

CHAPTER 9

Mental patients' rights
and legal redress

The law governing the practice of professionals (that is the law of tort)[1]
requires professionals to perform at a level considered to be reasonable. It
allows redress, usually in the form of financial compensation for those
harmed by failure to meet such standards. Lawyers would, I think, see the
law of tort as seeking to further three important social goals. First, it deters
socially undesirable conduct by forcing wrongdoers to pay the consequences, that is it operates as a deterrent and reduces the likelihood that
others will engage in such actions. Second, by transferring monies or some
other forms of compensation, justice (distributive justice that is) becomes
established. Third, the cost of successful actions means that if the defendant
has insurance – and in England and Wales that mostly means the
Medical Defence Union – the cost of these actions are not borne by him
alone but by all the policy holders. They in turn may be able to pass on the
increased costs of insurance to others. In this way policy holders and/or
customers collectively bear the cost of a predictable number of negligent
claims (Klein & Glover, 1983). To these three goals can be added a fourth:
that patients and psychiatrists alike know what can reasonably be expected
of them and know the acceptable standards.

For convenience, the rights of mental patients can be examined following
the thrust of the tort law generally. That is tort law covers injuries
negligently caused to patients, and injuries psychiatrists and others failed to
prevent through their own negligence. The former are more prosaic yet no
less important, the latter are more interesting and point to new areas of
development. The general point I wish to make is that legal barriers exist to
prevent the normal pattern of redress. In the second part of this chapter I

want to show that where those legal barriers have been removed, as under the 1983 Act, new possibilities exist to establish and promote patients' rights. Promotion of rights may, however, have certain unintended consequences.

To set the scene, remember that we are talking about 80000 beds in mental hospitals, or about 171 per 100000 of the population, or about 200000 admissions each year (Roth & Bluglass, 1985). To these should be added an unknown number of out patients, private or otherwise. Of the admissions, about 10% are compulsory under the 1983 Mental Health Act (formally under the 1959 Mental Health Act); the remainder can be called informal patients. It is with that smaller group of compulsory patients that this chapter is concerned.

Barriers against legal redress under earlier legislation

Traditionally, legal redress involves patients being able to establish that they have suffered physical or some other harm. Negligence occurs when practice falls below the accepted standards of professional competence and training (HMSO, 1978, para. 1308). The 1983 Act specifically grants certain rights to patients; it protects them from ill-treatment whether they be in hospital, or in the community as outpatients, or subject to guardianship (Section 127). It is an offence too for a man on the staff of a hospital or nursing home to have sexual intercourse with a woman receiving treatment, or with a woman on guardianship or otherwise in his custody. The patient is likewise protected against the forging of documents where the patient has been formally or compulsorily detained. Under the 1983 Act there are established rights preventing patients' mail being witheld or read (Section 134), and there are now rights to vote. There are rights too whereby detained patients can be informed of other rights such as access to Mental Health Review Tribunals. Some of these rights did not exist in earlier legislation and, in this respect, the 1983 Act is a step forward.

However, outside these specific areas matters are more cloudy; patients may find they are subject to the indignity of having personal belongings examined, day clothes may be taken away, and where compulsory detention may be translated as a general right on behalf of the hospital authorities to probe into all aspects of the patient's life. That many patients put up with this, and in an uncomplaining way, says much about the language and practice of medicine which has been able to assert dominance over the whole person, justified on the basis that actions will be in the patient's best interests. It says much too about modern psychiatric beliefs where challenges to professional dominance may be, and occasionally are, seen as subversive. Worse, they may be seen as being opposed to the interests of the patients generally, for they are seen as interrupting the therapeutic flow existing between the healers and the healed. Already a new term of abuse has begun to creep into the psychiatric literature, that of the 'libertarian' (Roth & Bluglass, 1985) seen as essentially disruptive, and anti-psychiatric. It is almost as if the high moral ground is being taken, where all are classified as being for psychiatrists or against them: libertarians are automatically seen as being in the opposing camp.

There are many areas, other than those mentioned above where patients' rights are uncertain, and many too where mental health legislation takes away rights unheard of in other areas of social life. The absence of appeal against a compulsory order being made, the manner in which patients can be transferred from an order of shorter duration to a longer one without appeal, the lack of precision in the legal terms governing admission are but further examples. The matter is not all one-sided: the right to detain informal mentally disordered patients wanting to leave hospital against advice places hospital staff in an invidious position although common law powers are said to exist (see Chapter 3).

In addition to those examples given above, mental patients are above all further disadvantaged by being unable to seek legal redress by the provision of Section 139 (formerly Section 141 of the 1959 Act). This section provides that, apart from proceedings against a health authority or the Secretary of State and those concerning the ill-treatment of patients (under Section 127) or other defined matters mentioned above, no civil or criminal proceedings can be brought against any person in any court in respect of an act done under the 1983 Act without the leave of the High Court or the Director of Public Prosecutions; for such proceedings to succeed, the Court must be satisfied that the person proceeded against acted in bad faith or without reasonable care.

There are many legal niceties relating to this section, making it difficult to determine what is an 'act purporting to be done in the persuance of mental health legislation'. It seems that agreement exists, as far as lawyers agree on anything that is, that it does not apply to informal patients, though it may do as far as the sections of the Act relating to consent to treatment are concerned. Agreement too exists that it applies to the general management of patients. This is a result of a House of Lords ruling in the case of Pountney v. Griffiths in 1976 (see Hoggett, 1984). There a nurse at Broadmoor was charged with common assault when he tried to return an unwilling patient to a different part of the hospital at the end of visiting time.

An earlier conviction by the magistrates was set aside by the Lords on the grounds that the nurse was acting in a manner purporting to be done in the pursuance of the legislation. This ruling shifted the emphasis, for the Percy Commission preceding the 1959 Act saw Section 141 as it then was as relating to the commitment procedure only. Agreement also exists that Section 141 does not apply to offences of ill-treatment and the like mentioned earlier, nor does it affect actions for *habeas corpus*. It could apply to prosecutions for acts done to those other than the patients: Hoggett (1984) gives the example of a hypothetical case where it was alleged a nurse had separated patient and family during a dispute at visiting time. In this instance the nurse could claim immunity.

Why introduce such legislation in the first place? There were two related reasons for this I think, both demanding a pragmatic solution to a complex problem. The first is that the State requires the Mental Health Acts to be operated and requires the cooperation of medical practitioners and others. They in turn argue that protection is needed if they are to avoid prosecution and be sued for honest mistakes. (No one suggests it should extend to malevolent practices.) The result first developed under the 1890 Lunacy Act was a *quid pro quo*. In order to obtain cooperation from the medical profession, and it was for the medical profession that protection was first granted, there had to be some degree of immunity (see further Bean, 1980). The 1890 Lunacy Act provided under Section 330(i) that medical men (and others) 'shall not be liable to any civil or criminal proceedings . . . if such persons have acted in good faith and with reasonable care'. There was a straightforward deal where the Lord Chancellor said if the medical profession wanted protection they had to take on board the certification procedure. The *British Medical Journal*(1889) said of the 1890 Act 'Though it satisfied no one and in many ways appears impracticable yet some legislation was longed for as a protection against medical men'.

As far as it went, the 1890 Act offered a reasonable compromise. Members of the medical profession, unlike say police are required to detain patients without the necessary legal training or available advice. Lacking legal protection they may refuse to operate the Acts lest they be open to vexatious litigation. (There was talk of strike action in 1885 when it was known that such legislation would be introduced.) As far back as 1885 Lord Coleridge said 'It would be lamentable if medical men were in such cases to be made responsible for honest mistakes'. His reasons for saying this would not I think be those advanced today for he said he feared that 'the consequences must be that those in the highest rank of their profession will refuse to sign certificates in lunacy cases and alleged lunatics be at the mercy of those at the lowest ranks' (quoted in Bean, 1980). Be that as it may, the problem highlighted by Lord Coleridge remains. Indeed in some countries the courts have held that psychiatrists who take part in commitment proceedings are to be immune from malpractice suits on the grounds that they, like judges, should be able to commit patients to mental hospitals without fear of liability. That is they are deemed to be acting in a judicial capacity. These decisions are interesting in their own right, tending to give support to theorists who see mental health legislation as an alternative control system (or at least as a parallel one operating adjacent to that of the criminal law).

The second reason is less credible in my view: it is that protection needs to be granted in order to prevent medical men being sued by vexatious litigants. Lord Simon in the judgment given above in the House of Lords said 'patients under the Mental Health Act 1959 may generally be inherently likely to harass those concerned with them by groundless charges and litigations, and may therefore have to suffer modifications of their general right of access to the courts' (quoted in Hoggett, 1984). There is no evidence to support this view, or at least he gave none, and much to suggest the contrary: that is mental patients are inherently passive, requiring other people to stand up for them. There are perhaps a few who are likely to be litiginous, but not many. As a group, mental patients may be no different than others, rather I would suggest that if anything they require as much or if not more protection than most.

It was however the 1959 Act that turned something reasonable into something more serious. The 1959 Act under Section 141 said 'No civil or criminal proceedings shall be brought against any person in any court in respect of any act without leave of the High Court, and the High Court shall not give leave under this Section unless there is substantial grounds for the contention that the person proceeded against has acted in bad faith and without reasonable care'. Notice that whereas the 1890 Act gave protection where such persons had acted in good faith and with reasonable care, a plaintiff had now to show that there existed bad faith and there was not reasonable care. An altogether more difficult task. Notice too that there had to be leave from the High Court, and the grounds had to be 'substantial'. So under the 1959 Act the wrong patient could be detained, the wrong documentation provided, the wrong diagnosis and treatment be given but the patient would have little redress unless there existed substantial grounds of bad faith and of a lack of reasonable care.

It is interesting to speculate on the reasons for such changes, especially as the 1959 Act also removed certification (that is the certificate of compulsory detention granted by the courts to detained patients). There was less opportunity to complain to any external body, and of course no right of appeal under the 1959 Act. A shift from legalism as a means of controlling the insane to a medical view produced more than a loss of procedural rules, it granted extended protection to the rule enforcers. The Percy Commission preceding the 1959 Act did not recommend such changes so we must look elsewhere for the reasons, and of course it comes as no surprise to see that very few applications for leave under Section 141 were granted: 4 in 1970, 1 in 1971, 3 in 1972, 7 in 1973 (5 by the same person) 4 in 1974, and 5 in 1975 (W. Bingley, personel communication).

It is also interesting to note that no member state of the Council of Europe, apart from those located in the British Isles, has legislative prohibitions similar to those of Section 141 of the 1959 Act. In Scotland and Northern Ireland access to the courts would be comparatively easier than in England and Wales or the Republic of Ireland. In Scotland there are no powers to seek leave prior to bringing proceedings, or to showing substantial grounds for the contention that the person to be proceeded against acted in 'bad faith' etc . . . The Scottish Act merely requires 'bad faith' and 'without reasonable care' as opposed to 'substantial grounds' (Section 122 of the Mental Health (Scottish) Act 1984). In Northern Ireland, legislation requires that leave must be obtained from a judge of the High Court of Northern Ireland who must be satisfied that there is a *prima facia* case. In the Republic of Ireland the Mental Treatment Act (Section 260) is in almost all respects similar to that of England and Wales suggesting a common legislative inheritance.

Considerable criticism has appeared over the years relating to Section 141 of the 1959 Act. Amendments have been introduced under the 1983 Act in Section 139 which, in general terms, do not amount to a great deal. They change the terms of the patient's burden of proof from 'substantial' to 'reasonable' grounds. Patients now require consent to be given for criminal proceedings by the Director of Public Prosecutions rather than the High Court who will, I understand, prosecute if there is a 50/50 chance of the prosecution succeeding. The High Court however will still deal with non-criminal matters and that Court will probably decide on the basis of a *prima facia* case – although Hoggett (1984) says it could just as easily be on the 'balance of probabilities'. She also says that even if the High Court decides on the basis of a *prima facia* case plaintiffs will still be at a disadvantage compared with other litigants. They will have to go first to a High Court judge whatever the size of their claim. They will have to verify the case by affidavit whereas most other litigants do not have to prove anything until the hearing. They will also run the risk that the judge considers their case bad on facts whereas other defendants can only escape by alleging that there is no cause of action in law. She makes the further point that it is difficult to know whether Section 139 as it now stands amounts to a denial of the plaintiff's right to have a fair and public hearing within a reasonable time by an independent and impartial court as required by Article 6(1) of the European Convention.[2] It could easily be a discrimination against him in the enjoyment of that right, contrary to Article 15.

However, there is a further important change in Section 139(4). This sub-section says 'This section does not apply to proceedings against the Secretary of State or against a health authority within the meaning of the National Health Service Act 1977' (notice that Local Authority Social Services Department are not listed with the Secretary of State or health authority). This change in conjunction with the reduction in the burden of proof referred to earlier is important as for the first time since 1890 it makes it easier for psychiatrists and other health authority employees to be sued through their Health Authority and brings mental disorders into the same position as medicine generally (see HMSO, 1978, ch. 24). Health authorities are vicariously liable for the actions of their employees and – as Health Authorities are likely to be worth more in financial terms than employees, whether covered by the Medical Defence Union or not – the possibilities are on the face of it extensive. In fact some lawyers are recognising them. So much so that organisations such as MIND have begun programmes protecting patients' rights in matters relating to the patients' deteriorating psychiatric condition, excessive use of ECT, sex hormone treatments, the over-prescribing or wrongful prescribing of drugs etc. MIND, like others entering this field must know they are entering a largely unchartered area where barriers exist other than formal ones. To name but a few there are the delays and costs of litigation, the difficulty in obtaining evidence, the difficulty of establishing causation, and that of quantifying damage.

Areas where litigation could be pursued under Section 139

Such changes in the legislation as have occurred fit into the general principles of tort law; that is citizens have rights to pursue actions for damages if there is a breach of statutory duty. Some critics would still argue that Section 139 does not go far enough but as the Parliamentary Debates show the government's view was that protection for those operating the Mental Health Act was still required (Parliamentary Debates, 4 March 1982). Of course the numbers and extent of actions where the Secretary of

State or the Local Health Authority will be proceeded against will be determined by a number of factors, not least the energy and competency of the legal profession linked to a similar sense of urgency from the patients. Hitherto patients' rights have been fashioned according to the demands of the medical professionals; increasingly demands of other professionals will define the area to be covered.

Assume that litigation will follow in the wake of the 1983 Act what are the likely areas open for development? It may be easier to say what is not, and to include those where doubts and uncertainties exist. Consent to treatment is already covered by the 1983 Act so, for these purposes, we can set that aside; so too are matters dealt with specifically under that Act such as ill-treatment of patients, sexual intercourse, rights to vote etc. It still remains unclear as to whether Section 139 applies to informal patients; some think so, others not. It is also unclear if Section 139 applies to the process of compulsory detention itself. Social workers are involved in the admission procedure and are employed by Local Authorities. The latter are not included in the exemption clause so that might complicate matters. There seems no reason why social workers should be exempt and one would hope that amendments to the 1983 Act, were there to be any would set aside this anomaly.

The case of Ashingdane v. UK (1983) brought before the European Commission of Human Rights would be permitted under the 1983 Act, but not under the 1959 Act. This application concerns the prolonged detention of the applicant in Broadmoor Special Hospital as of 1 March 1979 after he had been found fit for transfer to an ordinary mental hospital at Oakwood, Kent and the applicant's attempts to challenge the lawfulness of the authorities' refusal to transfer him. The transfer was made impossible by the refusal of the nurses trade union to accept patients like the applicant under Section 65 of the Mental Health Act 1959 on transfer from Broadmoor to ordinary mental hospitals which the nurses claimed had not the resources for dealing with such patients. The applicant complained to the Commissioner of his prolonged detention in Broadmoor and of the dismissal under Section 141 of the 1959 Act and of the action he brought against the Local Authority and the DHSS. He invoked Article 5 of the Convention, claiming that he was unlawfully detained not being a person of unsound nature whose compulsory detention in such conditions was necessary under Article 5(i) and alleging that he had no remedy under Article 5(4) by which the lawfulness of his detention could be determined. He also complained of a denial of access to a court in the determination of his civil rights, in breach of Article 6(1) of the Convention. Changes under the 1983 Act will mean that in future this type of case will presumably be dealt with locally in courts in England and Wales rather than by the European Commission.

It may also be possible that, under Section 139, claims of negligence can be pursued more vigorously than hitherto, as in those instances where psychiatric treatments were said to harm the patients. There are others, such as in cases of polypharmacy (which involve the concurrent use of several drugs) or where the use of major tranquillisers are maintained as matters of expediency rather than as part of a therapeutic programme. The prescribing of addictive drugs (such as barbiturates) may also be challenged if the drug dosage exceeds manufacturers' recommendations and guidelines when given to patients suffering from relatively minor psychiatric conditions. The psychiatrist may also be held strictly liable for a plaintiff's tardive dyskinesia, whether he was negligent or not.

Psychiatrists may also become liable for psychiatric patients who commit or attempt suicide. Klein & Glover (1983) say such cases as have been successful typically follow one of three basic patterns. Firstly psychiatrists are sued by surviving family members when a hospitalised patient commits suicide and where family members claim that adequate care and supervision had not been provided. Secondly where a psychiatrist is sued when a patient who was released from hospital commits suicide and the patient's family contend that the decision to release constituted negligence. And finally psychiatrists are sued when an outpatient they have been treating commits suicide. The plaintiffs claim that if the psychiatrist had provided adequate treatment the suicide would not have occurred. Psychiatrists may also be liable when a patient commits a violent act where it would be argued that the psychiatrist should have foreseen and prevented his patients' violent behaviour. Such actions have not been possible before, but as employers such as Area Health Authorities must vicariously accept liability for their employees then this new range of possibilities exists for detained patients.

Limitations and dangers in litigation

Before lawyers and patients relish too quickly their new-found freedom it is well to remember that in countries where litigation has traditionally been more open than in England and Wales (mainly in the USA) insurance premiums vary according to the nature of the medical specialism. Surgeons pay the highest, psychiatrists the lowest. This seems to reflect the state of market forces and if we assume that psychiatric patients are no more timid (in spite of what was said earlier) in the manner in which they approach litigation, then it seems reasonable to assume that differences are due to structural factors, such as the nature of the psychiatric specialism and the personal relationships contained therein. It may well be that the stigma attached to mental illness means that some patients fear the loss of privacy accompanying a lawsuit. Or, that patients often develop strong emotional ties to the psychiatrist which may make some patients reluctant to institute legal procedings. Finally, psychiatrists are trained in dealing with their patient's hostility and this may be able to forestall a threatened suit. Litigation, whether it be against the Area Health Authority or whatever, will never be an easy matter.

The Pearson Commission, concerned with compensation for personal injury, has provided the official statement on negligence.

The patients remedy at law is to sue his doctor for dangers. He must prove that, on the balance of probabilities the defendent was negligent. A doctor can clear himself if he can show that he acted within approved practice at the time the alleged negligence was caused. As Lord Clyde said 'To establish liability . . . where deviation from normal practice is alleged three facts are required to be established. First of all it must be proved that there is a usual and normal practice; secondly . . . that the defender has not adopted that practice; and thirdly (and this of crucial importance) . . . that the course the doctor adopted is one which no professional man of ordinary skill would have taken if he had been acting with ordinary care' (Hunter v. Hanley, 1955, S.C.200 at p. 206). It has been established that the doctor must take care to recognise a case which is beyond his skill, and refer it to another practitioner having the requisite skill.   HMSO (1976) para. 1309.

This statement by the Pearson Commission will form the basis of the subsequent discussion, although not necessarily in the order listed above.

Consider first the nature of the specialism, compared with other forms of medicine, say surgery for example. There is no central orthodoxy in psychiatry whether it be in the methods or types of treatment.[3] To ask of a psychiatrist the standard approach to this or that psychiatric condition is to ask a question which has less meaning than elsewhere in medicine. All specialisms are to some extent dictated by fashion but in most others fashions develop out of settled agreements about the basics and essentials. Not so in psychiatry. Types of treatment, even diagnosis, become associated with the personal beliefs of psychiatrists; leucotomies for example tended to be practiced by one or two psychiatrists (see Bridges, 1984) and it is still possible to hear of unmodified ECT being given and justified as a therapeutic technique (and by eminent psychiatrists). Equally there is no settled agreement on the forms of treatment to be given whether it be the types of drugs, the dosage, or the therapeutic milieu. That psychiatrist A relies heavily on Drug B for Condition C does not of itself tell us about standard practice; it says more of the therapeutic influences and personal experience of that practitioner. With little or no agreement in such matters it is not surprising that there is a lack of internal validity in the subject matter; this is reflected in the range of competing theories and claims. Where lawyers are unable to determine standard practices they are less likely to pursue successful claims of negligence or injuries occurring as a result of negligence. Elsewhere in medicine standard practices exist, providing a yardstick by which to measure substandard ones.

Perhaps plaintiffs may be more successful in matters relating to breaches of procedure that those involving treatment. By breaches of procedure I mean those where certain established routines exist, formally derived and governing such activities as the compulsory admission procedure, consent to treatment etc. Yet, here again, major problems must be overcome. The 1983 Act, like its predecessor, allows errors to be put right without affecting the status of the patient. Section 15(1) states, if within a period of 14 days the orders for commitment were found to be incorrect or defective, amendments may be made and those amendments 'shall have the effect as if they had been originally made as so amended'. Subsection 2 says that if a medical recommendation was faulty 'that medical recommendation shall be disregarded but the application shall be and shall be deemed always to have been sufficient . . .'. Faced with such a qualifying or let-out clause, errors of procedure (especially at the admission stage) are even more difficult to establish.

Similarly psychiatry, almost alone amongst branches of medicine, rarely initiates inquiries should things go amiss. The plaintiff, or his representative, therefore has no formal records from which to work, and must rely on the memory or goodwill of other staff members. The problems relating to this are not insurmountable but the advantages of being able to refer to written records of an inquiry are obvious, given the length of time taken to bring the case to hearing.

These apart, the central problem is to prove causation and proving causation in psychiatry is especially difficult. Three questions need to be asked. What are the results of treatment? What would happen if the patient had not received treatment? What would have happened if the patient had received a different treatment? In the first, types of treatment vary widely so that in psychotherapy for example the effects or impact of the therapist have to be disentangled from a host of intervening variables. To say that a patient suffered as a result of the psychotherapist rather than say another important figure in his life becomes quite difficult. In this, like all areas where psychiatry merges imperceptably with matters of personal relations, the results of one relationship cannot easily be separated from another. Where there is more direct intervention, say through drug therapy, the problems may be reduced and negligence more easy to establish. I am thinking here of the type of negligence where excessive doses of drugs have been prescribed, or where a sustained period of polypharmacy exists. Even so definitions of 'excessive' or 'sustained' are open to interpretation, dependent on other interpretations relating to the clinical definition of the patient, his previous history and the judgment of the psychiatrist.

In the second question, that is, what could have happened had the patient not received treatment, matters are no less easy. In medicine generally the natural history of the disease condition allows informed speculation on the likely consequences of leaving patients untreated. Not so in psychiatry, and for the reasons mentioned earlier. In the third question, that is what would have happened if the patient had received different treatment, there is the additional problem of having to evaluate the effects of another. Compare ECT with psychotherapy for example, or antidepressant A with antidepressant B. Given the problems surrounding the first and second questions, the third seems especially daunting.

Claims against negligent psychiatrists will, I suggest, never be easy and they are probably more difficult than elsewhere in medicine. Add to this the nature of the plaintiff (that is, plaintiffs who are mentally ill may make poor witnesses: they may be reluctant to place themselves in positions where they can be readily discredited, and where the nature of their illnesses makes it easy to discredit them further). Therefore to describe the task as 'daunting' is not hyperbolic. This on top of the problem of pursuing negligent claims where delays of 5 years are not unusual, where there are few specialist lawyers, and where there are few specialists prepared to be on the side of a plaintiff if it means being on opposite sides to a colleague. In such types of cases a GP's evidence is rarely acceptable, and specialists, outstanding in their field, are likely to be eagerly sought by the plaintiff and his opposite number. In negligence claims generally it has been estimated that only 1 in 50 reach a successful conclusion, so that compensation turns out to be more a lottery than a right. Road accident victims, for example, complain about the endless problems faced in finding a lawyer prepared to take their case, or worse still, finding themselves with an inexperienced one who gives up too easily or is prepared to accept too little compensation too quickly.

Translate the problems of negligent claims generally into that of the mental patients and the complexity and enormity of the task is obvious. 'Selling a dream' is how someone once put it. Add further that the mental patient is against the legal might and expertise of the Medical Defence Union – where, without legal aid, the initial costs can be prohibitive. Add also the prevailing attitudes of many members of the legal profession where mental patients may be regarded as a low-priority group, not the least because they will not command high compensation if as chronic patients their earning potential is low. 'Selling a dream' is not an exaggeration.

Perhaps I am being unduly pessimistic. Certainly the Medical Defence Union would think so. In their 1982 Annual Report they view the future with some alarm and urge medical practitioners to help 'stem the tide' of rising numbers of claims – not necessarily in the field of psychiatry, I would add. Various reasons are given for an increase in the number of claims: publicity surrounding large awards for damages is said to generate more claims, the assistance given to patients by pressure groups, the Limitation Acts which provide no protection against claims made outside the prescribed 3 year period, and high expectations of medicine where 'disappointment turns to bitterness and then into thoughts of litigation. In the old days when something went wrong in medicine . . . or if the ideal had not been achieved patients and their relatives generally took the attitude 'the doctors did their best, so its no ones fault, just bad luck'. Today the issues of fault or liability often predominates' (Medical Defence Union, 1982 p. 9).

There is not only the question of the limitations to consider for there are dangers too. Assume that mental patients are 'sold the dream' and find that, through Section 139(4), negligence claims can be made against Area Health Authorities, and hence against medical personnel. Assume too that mental patients are led to believe that obstacles can be overcome, what then? Will they generally be better off? Some say, if they can receive appropriate compensation but what of their contemporaries, and what of those who come after them? In principle, legal theorists suggest the social consequences of tort law will improve psychiatric practices and prevent rights being violated. Can we be certain of this? The answer I think must be equivocal for there may be unintended consequences which, in the long run, mean that certain rights become introduced, others established but others may be lost. Whatever the outcome I think we must proceed carefully. We must not enter blindly areas which are delicate at the best of times and rely on methods of cooperation between psychiatrist and patients which we hardly understand.

It has been assumed up until now that a vigorous pursuit of patients' rights, using traditions built up through the law of tort are automatically to the advantage of the patient. Ethically this is probably so, but there are other ethical questions to consider. How does the lawyer balance the right to compensation with the demands of the patient's health? Does he help the patient get better and risk losing a hefty compensation, or does he resist promoting rehabilitation until after the hearing? This ethical question is not peculiar to psychiatric patients but it exists nonetheless. Does the lawyer risk losing the goodwill of the patient's psychiatrist, the more so if the patient is long-stay and chronic, in the pursuit of the patient's rights? How will the patient withstand the lengthy delays before the final hearing, and what will be the effect if he is not successful?

What of the psychiatrists themselves? What will be the short-term and long-term effects on psychiatric practice? It is as well to remember that professional dominance exists, one effect of which is that psychiatrists can choose and select their patients. Assume for the moment that the position in England and Wales resembled that of the USA where Courts have been sympathetic to the claims that psychiatrists should be responsible for, and foresee and prevent patients' violent behaviour. When a psychiatric patient commits a violent act, in or out of the hospital, the victim of this violence will attempt to sue the psychiatrist. Ignore for these purposes other complexities involved such as those relating to psychiatric predictions of dangerousness, the duty to warn possible victims etc. and consider only the effect on psychiatric practice. Might it not be that psychiatrists will refuse to take such patients? If they did, would it be surprising? Given the demands to transfer as many people out of the Special Hospitals as possible, might not that expected trend be reversed? Certainly as Klein & Glover (1983) point out, the extent to which psychiatrists respond by refusing to treat potentially violent individuals will not reduce the incidence of violence. In their view, it may well increase it by leaving such individuals untreated or unattended.

Assume also that the courts in England and Wales are sympathetic to claims that where a patients committed suicide there remains a substantial risk of liability to the psychiatrist. Might not the effects be similar to those above; that is those patients who might commit suicide may be refused admission? More than that, and to quote Klein & Glover (1983) again, might the effect be perverse? That is, in order to avoid liability, psychiatrists become cautious. They may increase their supervision of patients and rely more extensively on chemical and physical restraints. They may also seek to delay the release of inpatients and hospitalise outpatients. If, as is generally believed, psychiatrists overpredict suicides then there may well be a tendency to extend supervision of inpatients and delay release. They may perhaps decide it is not worthwhile to attempt treatment anyway in which case some patients, not all by any means, may turn out have a higher risk of suicide than before.

Aside from these considerations, protection of mental patients rights raises interesting jurisprudential questions such as to what extent can anyone, psychiatrist or not, be responsible for the actions of another person, mentally ill or otherwise? To what extent can psychiatrists be expected to act the part of criminal prevention officer where offences are likely to be committed by patients on others? In addition there are more prosaic questions about the rights of mental patients generally, such as their rights to be free of psychiatric intrusion other than in specially defined treatment areas. There are also wider policy questions such as concern over the effect which legal determination of the rights of mental patients may have in resurrecting a new form of legalism. There are policy questions too about the introduction of a 'no-fault' scheme, as currently practised in New Zealand and Sweden. This was rejected by the Pearson Commission on numerous grounds (not least being the cost). There are problems of involving paramedicals such as nurses, physiotherapists etc. with such a scheme. Even so, the Commission recomended a no-fault scheme should be 'studied and assessed so that the experience can be drawn upon if because of changing circumstances a decision is taken to introduce a 'no-fault' scheme for medical accidents in this country' (HMSO, 1978, para. 1371). If so, what are the implications of all this? These questions will need to be raised when litigation is extended through Section 139. My concern here has been more limited: to document and examine the issues at a more restricted level, recognising that in this early stage questions need to be asked rather than answers provided.

CHAPTER 10

The effectiveness of legal rights

In England and Wales we have pursued vigorously a campaign aimed at promoting legal rights for mental patients. The 1983 Act was the apotheosis of that. Some commentators have referred to the Act as a return to legalism defined as the control of mental patients by the rule of law and its accompanying regulations. This description of the 1983 Act is somewhat hyperbolic; it would be more true to say that some imbalances have been redressed and occasionally tipped in favour of the mental patient by reducing the discretion granted hitherto to the professionals. The method directed towards limiting discretion has been fashioned in the idiom of patients' rights, where rights are defined as the ability or power to alter existing legal arrangements and to impose on others a duty to accept those arrangements.

This is not to say that earlier legislation ignored the question of rights, rather that the rights granted were of the wrong sort. Rights under the 1959 Act, (and, for these purposes, we are talking of patients' rights as opposed to the rights of medical staff) were tied up with treatment, a right which appeared to dominate all else. The right to receive treatment implied a duty on the psychiatrist to provide the treatment. It followed therefore that decisions about treatment had to be placed in the hands of the professionals. The model of the physician/patient relationship was transferred to mental patients but with the added twist that mental patients were definitionally unable to make decisions for themselves. The result, under the earlier 1959 Act was paternalism. It was a reaction to that which helped produce its 1983 counterpart.

It is interesting to see how some critics of the 1983 Act hark back to earlier days and hail the 1959 Act as a piece of liberal legislation or, as Sir Martin

Roth calls it, 'the century's most humane piece of legislation in relation to the mentally ill to be placed on the statute books anywhere' (Roth, 1985, p. 1). Of course there were advantages for the patient, but the 1959 Act was certainly not liberal, unless liberalism is defined as providing a one-sided set of freedoms for those who enforce the rules, and a duty to obey from the patients. It is interesting too that the relationship between law and psychiatry was also seen in rosier terms than today. Sir Martin Roth (1985) believes that under the 1959 Act there were great prospects for a close understanding between law and psychiatry, a relationship said to be full of high promise. Yet lawyers had very little to do with earlier mental health legislation. There was no interprofessional understanding as such: psychiatrists were given a free rein and lawyers let them get on with it. Matters changed when lawyers, or at least one or two of them, began to take an interest in mental health legislation, subjecting it to legal scrutiny and canons of natural justice. In doing so they found it wanting. After the 1983 Act Sir Martin Roth (1985, p. 8) talks of a rift arising between law and psychiatry and an estrangment between the two professionals. The rift was, I suggest, an inevitable outcome of legal involvement. He seems not to recognise the growth of a civil rights movement generally where mental patients have been swept into that movement and, in some instances, become the focal point of it.

Certainly the thrust towards patients' rights has become a guiding slogan of the early 1980s. One effect has been to force the lawyer into prominence. If there is such a rift, and I believe there is, the gap will not be bridged by a greater understanding of the various professional tasks, for law and psychiatry stem from different epistemological traditions. One emphasises the rational self-determination of the individual, the other the deterministic nature and effects of the disease condition. One starts from the assumption that legal rules protect patients from arbitrary decisions, the other that rules inhibit and restrict treatments. One sees the vagueness of psychiatric definitions as an indication of loose thinking, the other that tight definitions based on a type of internal validity mask the complexities of the human condition. At the level of practice, psychiatrists complain that lawyers have neither clinical responsibility nor experience of patient care. It is not then that lawyers do not understand psychiatry, say the psychiatrists, but that, ascribing themselves the patients' guardians, lawyers remain on the sidelines, avoid detailed patient contact yet claim to represent their interests. In return lawyers see psychiatrists as unable to accept that lawyers have traditionally claimed to be guardians of all liberties, for mental patients or otherwise. So the arguments go on.

Certainly lawyers seem to have taken and held the high moral ground with psychiatrists being placed on the defensive. How quickly fortunes change. In the late 1960s and early 1970s psychiatry promised everything – whether it be through insights gained by psychotherapy or by technical achievements through the pharmacological revolution. Psychiatrists were given the power to transmit those promises into action. Now things are different. Psychiatrists must forever justify themselves and are forced to give reasons for their decisions, whether they be for admissions, types of treatment or continued detention. Yet it seems reasonable to ask if greater legal involvement will produce the necessary benefits, or will patients swap one professional tyranny for another? At this stage the answer is far from clear. Legal intervention may promote worthwhile changes in psychiatric practices, yet it may also promote dissatisfaction. The latter may be based on a belief that legal rights offer protection against all perceived misdemeanors, and a belief that lawyers will remain on hand to give that protection. In all this however we sometimes forget the patients themselves. We cannot assume, as some lawyers and others do, that all patients may welcome more rights. Some may not. Some may be indifferent, or see rights as acting against their best interests. Indifference may be a product of cynicism or an unwillingness to be involved in matters outside the purely psychiatric sphere, or a belief in the irrelevance of rights, or perhaps even a view that an assertion of rights may create displeasure amongst the hospital staff. Some may believe or think that rights movements are misdirected or wrong in principle because they reduce the quality of care or intrude in the relationship between psychiatrist and patient. They may see rights activists and rights movements generally as affecting the proper order of things. Mostly they may see rights as nothing more than another set of hindrances which neither interests them nor which they wish to understand. It remains an all-too-common fallacy to think that because I or others believe something to be good, and believe it to be good for people generally it will be accepted as such.

Mental patients' rights

It is not necessary to list all the criticisms of the earlier 1959 Act related to patients' rights but some can be given. For example there were no provisions for consent to treatment whether for compulsory or informal patients. That is, patients had neither the choice nor a say in the method and types of treatment given (which could range from relatively benign forms of psychotherapy to irreversible and less benign forms of brain surgery). There was no real choice granted to patients concerning admission, nor could there be as long as there existed the threat of formal controls. There was no right of appeal prior to admission and limited appeals procedures thereafter. For informal patients, there was a right to be discharged but this right was far from certain when other legal controls existed which could override it. There was no right to privacy once inside the hospital; personal belongings could be systematically checked and searched and contents temporarily confiscated. There was no general right to legal redress for, in most instances, patients had to go to the High Court and show that the act in question was done in bad faith or without reasonable care. Conversely, there was a right granted to the hospital authorities to have powers of control and discipline over all their patients. In practice however the extent of such controls were less than clear. Some legal theorists saw them as 'similar to those enjoyed by the master of a ship' to use Glanville Williams phrase, others as governed by the concept of reasonableness, to use that of Hoggett (1984, p. 205).

I mention these criticisms, not just to go over ground covered in earlier chapters but to illustrate numerous areas where patients' rights were said not to exist – or rather not to any degree – and illustrate too that the 1983 Act has dealt with some but not others. It has, for example, dealt with consent but provided nothing in the form of an appeal procedure prior to admission. It has provided partial relief for those seeking legal redress in the courts but nothing about the rights to privacy. In this respect the movement towards patients rights has been selective, emphasising some, ignoring others, and – if the truth be known – taking some away which existed before (though this may not be the fault of individual rights activists but a means by which governments balance competing demands from various interest groups). Of course, no government could be expected to deal with everything and the introduction of the Mental Health Act Commission provides an overarching forum where rights are expected to be promoted generally (the activities of the Commission will be dealt with later in this chapter). Even so, one looks in vain for any systematic approach towards patients rights from those most closely involved. Many, whose claim it was to raise issues relating to rights, have not tended to promote a coherent rights programme. Rather they have produced something more akin to an *ad hoc* response emphasising certain features and neglecting others. I am not criticising these achievements, merely contrasting the success gained in some areas with the neglect of others.

To speak of an *ad hoc* response is perhaps to be unfairly critical for the activities of one or two campaigners stand out as providing a degree of consistency. Larry Gostin, for example, as legal officer of MIND alerted many (including those in government) to a large number of the more glaring defects of earlier legislation. As a key figure working for the foremost British pressure group in the mental health field, an examination of his activities linked to pressure group theory would repay careful study. Even so Gostin sometimes appears to have promoted or rather emphasised certain rights on the basis of his personal knowledge of and affection for countries elsewhere. He has, after all, consistently pushed a North American view whether it be in matters of consent or what he calls 'the ideology of entitlement' (see Chapter 5). A study of the interplay between his campaigns and the government's response is yet to be written but, when it is, it may explain the manner in which certain rights were accepted and others given less prominence.

Aside from this there is the question of the philosophical basis on which some of the rights campaigns were projected. Rarely did it appear that rights were being promoted according to a defined social theory unless attempts to compare existing legislation with principles of common law constitute such a theory. Yet all too often this seemed to be the favoured legal approach where, if existing legislation was held to violate common law principles, the argument was seen to be concluded: violation of common law was held to be self-evidently wrong and legal amendments required accordingly (see particularly Lanham, 1974). The debate more often than not failed to get beyond this.

Sometimes too it appeared that campaigners promoting rights were almost asserting a natural rights argument, or at least coming close to it. I say this because claims were often made as if they were self-evident truths based on a set of *a priori* assumptions. Claims for property rights and for the preservation of certain freedoms are cases in point. They were presented as rights not to be pushed aside for the sake of interest groups or the pursuit of other social goals and aspirations. These rights, it was asserted, were to be protected by governments for they were attached to and could be claimed by everyone whatever and wherever their situation. It mattered not that mental hospital authorities might wish to assist, or even bring about a cure of their patients, rights must prevent certain forms of intervention irrespective of the honourable intentions of those who would intervene.

The first and most obvious problems of these types of campaigns is (again) that of the demand for a theory. Even in the liberal tradition some philosophers have insisted that rights could be taken seriously only if they were understood as being based on *a priori* theory of social morality. What is often infuriating about exponents of the common law arguments or the natural-rights-type argument is that a theory seems not to exist. The idea that those rights could be a starting point for any form of political morality – which, for these purposes, means psychiatric morality – was and would have been regarded by some, notably Jeremy Bentham as wild and pernicious nonsense. Others have been equally appalled that rights can be claimed and interests asserted against the community. Or, as Marx said, 'none of the so called rights of man goes beyond egoistic man . . . [of] an individual withdrawn behind his private interests and whims and separated from the community' (quoted in Waldron, 1983, pp. 1–2). I am not asking that modern lawyers concerned with patients rights had to be grounded into one theory (in his case, utilitarianism). I am nonetheless concerned that most lawyers have failed to consider any theory at all, except to raise the spectre of the common law, which is at best a starting point for a theory rather than a conclusion.

The second problem, and related to the first is that assertions derived from common law allow few connections to be made with the aims or objects of the social tasks. That is, rights have been asserted or claimed sometimes with no thought or consideration for the social setting in which they exist, and this seems to be what Marx meant when he saw them related to 'egoistic man'. To claim for example the right of privacy in a mental hospital may affect seriously the smooth running of the mental hospital, may curtail effective treatment and allow individual patients to be unnecessarily disruptive. (I am not saying it would, merely using privacy as example of what could happen, although as will be argued later the opposite could equally be true namely that the ascription of rights has less effect on the quality of patient care than may be supposed.) There was little in the campaigning literature of the 1983 Act concerned with the effect of imposing rights in institutions such as mental hospitals, or any attempt to relate the effects of those rights to patient care generally. Again, it was almost as if the argument stopped at the point where the common law was violated and so by implication, and definitionally, breaches of common law must be rectified.

The exception was the MIND campaign with its chief advocate Larry Gostin. Here it was possible to identify a more consistent approach where the aim was to promote patients' rights on the model of equity. That is mental patients ought not to be deprived of certain rights because they were mental patients. So for example mental patients ought not to be deprived of a right to vote which was granted to others, they ought not to be deprived of consent to treatment which was granted to patients in other hospitals, they ought not to be deprived of rights of privacy which were granted elsewhere (and so on and so on). What Gostin and MIND did was to show how the

1959 Act had taken away the rights of mental patients, in comparision with other groups, and demanded their return. It was an effective campaign and one which was worthy of support. Its achievements were immense and could be said to have changed the face of mental health legislation in England and Wales and in Britain generally.

Even so, some of the criticisms applied to other campaigns could be directed towards that of MIND. It lacked a social theory except that of equity which is largely a legal theory; it paid little attention to the effects of rights on the objects of the social task, and lacked any attempt to relate those campaigns to the effect on patient care. It was also opportunistic – and again I say this without wishing to be critical or dissociate myself from that campaign. Its opportunism stemmed from its willingness to make application to the European Court as and when it suited. In many of Larry Gostin's writings (see particularly Gostin 1979) he compares mental health legislation in England and Wales on the basis of the yardstick of the common law and finds it wanting. One would have thought then that the common law, itself a developing and growing phenomenon would have been the vehicle for the campaign but MIND used the European Court instead. That court operates within a different legal tradition starting from a set of *a priori* assumptions formulated into a Bill of Rights. The judges are drawn from the member states having little or no experience of the social situation in England and Wales yet capable of making legal pronouncements which must be accepted, given Britain's membership of the European Community. A number of judgments made as a result of legal representation by MIND had to be included in the 1983 Act (one of which led to changes in Tribunal procedure). These were all to the good in one way, and more so if one happens to agree with that judgment but differing legal traditions tend to make unhappy bedfellows. I think we have not heard the last of that by a long way.

In all this we ought not to forget the role of the government. The government accepted the European Court's decisions, accepted too some campaign demands but did nothing about others. If one looks closely at the 1983 Act, it offered many of the advantages of a reforming piece of legislation but had the additional advantage of costing the government little – with the exception of the Mental Health Act Commission. Perhaps this accounted for the success of some of the campaigns. The government had earlier stated it had no wish to alter the premises on which mental health legislation had existed, rather it wanted to tidy up existing anomalies. On this basis then, translating common law rights or whatever into legislation became a neat, though limited, way of dealing with matters. Rights, of the common law type, could be inserted without raising fundamental questions, and introduced without changing central philosophies. Or, and perhaps more important, without costing money. Patients could be granted rights, in a positive sense of the term, and duties imposed on the treatment officials leaving other matters as before. If I am correct about this, then it was almost as if a functional dependency existed between the government and the legal campaigners where one was wishing to accept limited change the other providing the impetus. What more convenient way then to resurrect common law principles if the object is to leave the *status quo* intact or promote changes which cost little in additional funds. This is perhaps an overstatement but, given the climate under which the 1983 Act was introduced, not perhaps a gross overstatement and certainly a point worth considering in any detailed examination of the way the 1983 Act was promoted.

Rights as forms of social change

By implication the introduction and presence of patients' rights suggests some form of social change, whether as a means of promoting development or preserving a *status quo*. The question then is to what extent have rights and, particularly those inserted in the 1983 Act, promoted change and to what extent are those changes desirable? The latter of course depends on one's normative position.

Logically all rights imply duties. If a patient has a right to leave a hospital, the psychiatrist and staff have a duty to act with forebearance. If a patient has a right to be given certain types of treatment, it becomes the duty of those to provide him with it. If a patient has a right to privacy, there is a duty on others not to invade that privacy, and so on. Rights for these purposes are claim rights so that where rights are violated we say the bearer has been wronged. He can demand its performance and is entitled to demand that others act on his behalf (Waldron, 1984). Duties, on the other hand, are those acts which one is bound by an obligation to do. They may involve not doing something (as where the patient may exercise his right to leave hospital) or they may involve something more active where there is a right to treatment; sometimes they involve a mixture of both (as with the patients right to privacy). Even so, assume that rights are good, and assume too a more active involvement from the patient; what happens then? Let us posit the existence of a mental hospital where patients' rights cover various aspects of the patient's hospital career, such as admissions, treatments or discharge. Assume too that staff and patients are aware of those rights and there is a Board or Commission or something of similar standing ready to enforce them. Assume also that the staff have no wish to remove those rights or violate them. Could it then be guaranteed that the quality of patient care will improve as a direct result of those rights?

As far as rights enacted under the 1983 legislation the answer is probably not. Here the prevailing pattern of rights are of the more negative form; that is they are aimed at stopping intervention. They do so by restricting the powers of the hospital staff through the use of certain types of treatments without consent, by providing access to Mental Health Review Tribunals (MHRTs), by preventing sexual abuse by staff, by preserving interests in patients' property etc. In so doing they again draw on the tradition of the common law, but add that of the negative libertarians. In the latter the aim is to guard that minimum area of personal freedom deemed necessary for patients to exist without experiencing excessive intervention. The two traditions (common law and negative liberty) have much in common and sometimes appear indistinguishable. They both recognise the value of liberty and accept it as self-evidently so, and both see frontiers, not artificially drawn within which men should be inviolable, these frontiers being defined in terms of rules so long and widely accepted that their observance has entered into that conception of what it is to be a human being (Berlin, 1969, p. 165). Preservation of these frontiers has little or nothing to do with patient care *per se*, it being more important to protect patients against excessive forms of intervention. Of course some more positive benefits may accrue, but that is not necessarily the aim. The major aim is different; it is to allow the individual that level of personal freedom, in order to remain an individual. It is an attack on all those who preceded and supported the Comptian view, or rather the question Comte asked. 'If we do not allow free thinking in chemistry or biology why should we allow it in morals or politics (or psychiatry even)?' Why indeed? One either shares Comte's view or not. For my part I agree with Isaiah Berlin who cannot accept that there can in principle be only one correct way of life; that the wise lead it spontaneously that is why they are called wise. The unwise must be dragged towards it by all the social means in the power of the wise, lest demonstrable error be allowed to survive and breed (Berlin, 1969).

To return to that hypothetical mental hospital where rights are protected and preserved: it is possible under these circumstances for the treatment staff to be autocratic, despotic and unconcerned with the quality of patient care but (provided they do not violate patients rights) they could easily meet with approval. They may have little interest in patient care, may even have a low opinion of their patients but still be acceptable as preservers of rights.

This is I think the basis of criticisms of some rights movements generally where patients are said to be 'dying with their rights on'. The quality of care appears to matter little as long as rights are preserved.

Under the 1983 Act matters are a good deal more complicated than this and that hypothetical hospital must remain at that level. Not all rights remain in the form of negative liberty so described. Some, though they may have their origins in negative liberty and more directly in the common law, can promote change, even if not intentional. Consent procedures for example, as currently framed in the 1983 Act can reduce idiosyncratic decisions and place existing practices under greater scrutiny. By insisting patients be discharged from secure hospitals, MHRTs may force governments to provide alternative facilities. Rights can help patients change existing practices by promoting a new view of themselves: perhaps unintentionally. They maybe seen in a more circumscribed manner than hitherto, even commanding more respect. Those whose duty it is to protect these rights will recognise the limitations imposed on their powers and be affected accordingly. At the policy level when new procedures are developed and implemented, there must be accomodation to structural changes. Officials whose duty it is to protect rights (such as lawyers, or members of the Mental Health Act Commission) must also be accomodated and become less of an intruder in a world from which they were earlier excluded. Sometimes this is no small matter for one or two members of the Mental Health Act Commission have stated publicly (MIND Conference, March 1965) that, in its early days, some psychiatrists refused to see Commissioners, resenting the intrusion and challenges to their clinical judgments. It seems reasonable to suppose therefore that legal rights for mental patients produce ripples of change within the institutional settings – perhaps irrespective of the direct activities of the patient.

Yet, set against this, are a further set of practical difficulties. The manner in which modern rights are enacted provides rules which not only require enforcement but require knowhow and access to the rights-enforcing institutions. Mental patients, often due to the nature of their condition, may be unaware of their rights or for other reasons be unable to assert their rights as often as others are able to. They require assistance, mostly from outside bodies or representatives. Mental hospitals, and that includes many other areas covered by mental health legislation operate away from public scrutiny. This would not be a problem in that hypothetical hospital, but the real world is not always like that. Hospital staff may fail to protect rights, whether from ignorance or malevolence. Ignorance may stem from not knowing the rules (and many hospital staff appear not to; see Bean, 1980);

malevolence may occur when rights are seen to interrupt treatment or are perceived as anti-therapeutic in some way. Unlike rights which exist in the courts, there is rarely an opportunity to scrutinise methods of practice, or to cross-examine witnesses formally. We cannot assume that those working with mental patients will always be above reproach.

As a method of promoting social change, rights are of limited value. On the one hand they can improve the patients perception of himself, prevent intrusion and, perhaps, set standards. On the other they rarely promote new, more humane, and perhaps even more efficient methods of handling patients. The reason I suggest is not too difficult to see: patients' rights and patient care stem from different sources. There is one view that man should be protected from those who could care for him, for all are prone to abuse him. The other view suggests that patient care deals with the whole person and requires direct intervention in aspects of his life. The former can be traced to a Kantian view that paternalism is the greater evil, or to Mill where the sovereignty of the individual is paramount, the latter from a view that mental illness is debilitating and to cure the patient becomes an ethically justified task. Hence we return again to the differences between law and psychiatry and the different epistemological traditions, adding perhaps somewhat wryly that Sir Martin Roth's plea for understanding between the two disciplines is more likely to show that they talk past each other rather than make contact.

The effectiveness of rights in the 1983 Act

The old Board of Control (its predecessor was the Commission in Lunacy) had duties derived almost entirely from the Lunacy and Mental Treatments Acts 1890 and 1930 and the Mental Deficiency Act of 1913. With the introduction of the National Health Service (NHS), the Minister of Health became responsible for the control and supervision of local authority services and of NHS hospitals, as well as registration and licencing of hospitals outside the NHS. The Board of Control was responsible for matters affecting the patients and their rights. It was not always clear who was responsible for what, as questions of hospital policy could not easily be separated from those of the interests of the patients. Even so, the system worked reasonably well. The Board's powers were however largely advisory whereas the NHS commissioners were a more powerful body. The Percy Commission favoured the abolition of the Board of Control, thanking them for their sterling work over the years but finding no place for them in the new scheme of things. There was no equivalent Board for other areas of medicine and, as psychiatry was to become more integrated into medicine generally, the Board was an anomaly. The Percy Commission represented a new era, the old one was to pass for ever, or so it was thought. Many commentators agreed: they saw the abolition of the Board as a welcome step, believing that psychiatry could be integrated more fully under one Minister for Health. The Percy Commission went further: it saw the Board providing a system of control which was outdated and unnecessary. Moreover, as at least half the members of the Board were not medical practitioners they could not, according to the Percy Commission be expected to pronounce on medical matters. So, under the 1959 Act, the Board of Control ceased to exist leaving the Health Service Commissioner as the only watchdog.

It is a little surprising then that a Mental Health Act Commission should be introduced under the 1983 Act, and equally surprising that it was proposed by the Royal College of Psychiatrists, who expressed regret about the demise of the old Board – although as the Board of Control had few direct powers, the Royal College was likely to be more enthusiastic about a duplicate than a patient-advocacy scheme suggested elsewhere. Of course Commissions themselves tend to be unwieldy institutions. One could even describe them as lumbering compared to an adversarial system which offers a direct method followed by the maximum publicity. It was also surprising, given the experience of the Commission in Scotland, which has existed since 1960, and a vigorous one at that, making 'it hard to understand why the Scots were thought to need such an informed and caring body while the English and Welsh were not' (Hoggett, 1984, p. 219).

The Commission was introduced under Section 120 of the 1983 Act and described by the Secretary of State for Social Services as the 'single most important innovation in the Act'. Moreover 'it would carry on where Parliament leaves off' (Parliamentary Debates, 22 March 1982). Officially the Commissioners' tasks are

. . . to make themselves available to detained patients who ask to see them, and ensure that staff are helping patients to understand their legal position and their rights. They will look at patients records of admission and renewal of detention and at records relating to treatment. They will also ensure that detained patients are satisfied with the handling of any complaints they make.   DHSS (1980).

The Commission has six major functions: (*a*) appointing medical practitioners and other persons for the purposes of providing a second opinion and verifying matters relating to consent; (*b*) receiving and examining reports on treatment given under those consent provisions; (*c*) keeping under review the exercise of the powers and the discharge of the duties conferred or imposed by the Act relating to the detention of the patients or those liable to be detained; (*d*) proposing to the Secretary of State codes of practice related to matters contained in the Act; (*e*) to review censorship in the Special Hospitals; and (*f*) publishing a report every second year which must be laid before Parliament.

The Commission itself is a peculiarly British solution – though perhaps hardly fair to Scotland which has a superior system in that respect. It has all the hallmarks of a decisive thrusting body but its powers, composition and approach render it less than that. It was almost as if the government was fearful of going too far along a path which would offend professional bodies and so held back at the crucial moment. If so, then this was surely an error, for once the Commission loses its respect as a hard-hitting independent body it will find difficulty in being recognised as the protector of patients' rights.

Consider first its powers, or rather consider the powers it doesn't have. It doesn't have powers to deal with the informal patients who constitute about 90% of the hospital population. There are under Section 121(4) powers to deal with such patients but the Government has said that it does not intend to invoke those powers, for the Commission's first priority must be the detained patients. In practice then a very large number of patients lie outside the Commissions remit. This could of course be remedied later, the more so as the truly vulnerable are the younger mentally impaired or the elderly psychogeriatric patients. These are rarely detained compulsorily. It doesn't have powers to insist on hospital staff helping Commission members or providing them with documents in the manner of the Ombudsman, and it lacks the power of the Health Service Commissioner to compel the attendance of witnesses and receive information on oath. It doesn't provide patients with the right of access to their medical records. It doesn't have powers to deal with recalcitrant hospitals who refuse to acknowledge the adverse consequences of their actions or to correct them. It doesn't have powers to enforce codes of practice. These codes must remain at the level of a set of proposals – and described as being similar to the Highway Code (Rassaby & Rassaby, 1985).

There is the matter of the composition of the Commission. It consists of a Chairman and 90 members appointed by the Secretary of State and chosen from the legal, medical, nursing, psychology and social work professions together with a group of lay people with a special interest in the subject ('the wise and the good'). The Commissioners are appointed for 2–4 years; their appointment may be renewed on expiration, and they work 1–1½ days per week. The general consensus seems to be that appointments were safe in the sense that ardent and provocative campaigners were omitted, there were no patients or ex-patients on the Commission and those appointed were described by Alan and Elaine Rassaby (1985) as 'prominent well connected individuals' implying that the members were slightly out of touch with the mainstream of social life.

Aside from the personal composition of the Commission there are the structural features to consider. The Commission is appointed by the Secretary of State for Social Services and is subject to his directions. Rassaby & Rassaby (1985) describe it as 'a quasi-independent departmental complaints body' and they further state that 'the Commission must be conscious of the need to win the confidence of the Secretary of State and hospital staff by measures which are sufficiently cautious to avoid wounding the sensibilities of a conservative medical and nursing profession. Clearly the Commission is the gift of the Secretary of State; its report is presented through him rather than direct to Parliament or through a Select Parliamentary Committee. The manner in which the two major functions of the Committee (its planning and investigative functions) are within the same rubric of appointment, compromises the second and aims to please with the first. This all weakens or lowers its general credibility.

Little of this would be important if the methods adopted by the Commissioners appeared to suggest a more robust approach rather than a gentlemanly or conciliatory one. For example, the Commissioners will withhold records from patients if instructed to do so by the responsible medical officer, hospitals are notified of an impending visit (permitting what some critics call 'opportunities for spring cleaning') and there is no inclination to publicise issues, or to name publicly recalcitrant hospitals. Indeed the whole approach seems to be one which attempts to resolve conflicts in a manner which appears to avoid direct confrontation. If this is so then one ought not to be surprised if the patients believe that the Commission is not on their side but on that of the authorities. It is I think interesting to note that of a sample of complaints presented to the Commisson between 30 September 1983 and 22 January 1985 (during its first 18 months) hospital staff who are potentially a large source of complaint played no part in initiating complaints to the Commission. One can interpret this in a number of ways: either the staff see nothing about which to complain, or they have closed ranks to protect themselves, or they do not believe the Commission is likely to grant anonymity, or they have little faith in the Commissioner's ability to deal adequately with matters. If the reason for their lack of complaints is the last, then things are very serious indeed.

What then is the Commission likely to achieve in the patients' rights field? The answer must lie within the Commission's defined methodology; that is within the parameters of a conciliatory approach where the aim is to pursuade, to ease and to move people gently in certain directions. It cannot therefore expect success with persistent recalcitrant hospitals but it may push the more amenable in the required direction. It may also help set standards by easing psychiatrists towards more acceptable forms of treatment achieved through conciliation, discussion and example. What it ought not to do is create a climate whereby the Commission becomes the sole forum for debate. This would mean waiting until the Commission made its pronouncements which would then be translated into the Commission's language. In that way the Commission would be the centre of all authority and rather than encouraging debate may tend to stifle it. The dangers of producing a large centralised authority required to produce annual reports etc. is that little else happens without direct reference to it.

An assessment of the rights movement

The history of mental health legislation over the last century in England and Wales has been directed towards balancing sets of competing claims: those relating to the demands of treatment and those of patients' rights. Prior to the 1959 Act when the dominant theme was legalism which involved the courts in all matters relating to admissions to mental hospitals; the obvious advantage was to preserve rights and to defend legal procedures. The obvious defect was to delay treatment until the courts had adjudicated. Moreover, in spite of elaborate legal rules the courts were largely influenced by the opinions of the medical practitioners. Then came the 1959 Act and with it the dominance of the medical paradigm. As a result the courts faded into the background.

The 1959 Act dispersed power among the medical profession and, to a lesser extent, to social workers and allied medical services. Parallels with the juvenile justice system are instructive where social workers were granted powers under the 1969 Children and Young Persons Act which had hitherto been the province of the juvenile court. There, as in mental health legislation, came a recognised need to retrieve that power without returning to earlier legislative forms. In practice, retrieval meant finding ways of restricting professional activities and limiting the professionals role. The rights movement in mental health also attempts this. Elsewhere, and in the juvenile justice system, the children's rights movement tries to do likewise except that it has had a less formal tradition than that in mental health. In juvenile justice, controls have been more diverse; the Courts have had some powers returned to them, social work case conferences and formal panels have been diluted by the appointment of independent members, and so on (see for example Adoption Regulations 1983). In mental health the whole commitment has been towards changes in legislation, and less towards direct involvement in the daily management of patients through committees or official panels – with the exception of the Mental Health Act Commission.

This approach, which relies heavily on formal legal rules rather than diluting power through the committee or panel method, makes mental health rights a largely passive affair. It relies heavily on a legal interpretation of rights being devised by lawyers with legal definitions in mind. It operates according to what I have called legal theory where legal rules are introduced and lawyers and others wait for those rules to be broken. They then rail against the misuses (Bean, 1985); this is not entirely the case but it occurs sufficiently often to permit such a generalisation to be made. It relies on patients and others defining their rights according to the law and seeking professional legal assistance when those rights have been unlawfully violated. It relies too on active involvement by lawyers eager to take up the patient's cause.

This approach has many advantages. It introduces a belief that mental patients are more than the aggregate of their psychiatric symptoms and forces attention on the way in which patients are viewed, in mental hospitals or elsewhere. It creates an impression that patients are neither wholly mad nor wholly sane but in the midst of their insanity can be presumed to be capable of making decisions. It protects their self and their essential humanity. It controls, or exerts pressure on the maverick psychiatrist bringing him into line with more realistic psychiatric thinking. It requires all patients be they in Special Hospital or elsewhere to have their case considered regularly at a formal level. It does all this and much more. It does not help answer other basic questions. It cannot go beyond legal thinking and consider other policy questions which loom in importance. It cannot do this because it was not intended to move in that direction. The intention was always to act as a brake on excessive psychiatric powers.

Its success or failure should however be evaluated according to its restricted aims. The activities of one organisation such as MIND could never be expected to achieve more than limited results. That the MIND campaign broke the mould of the past, that it helped change attitudes, help shift views and ask questions hitherto unasked guarantees its success and its place in psychiatric history. But the mental patients' rights movement, as currently constructed, should I think be seen as a phase in a longer stage of development, and a phase which was welcomed by a government which found that mental patients' rights (in the manner instituted) had a certain populist appeal yet cost little in additional expenditure. Those involved in the campaign leading to the 1983 Act may not have seen it that way but I think this is what happened. The more interesting question now seems to be 'where next?'

One possibility is to produce more of the same. It was said above that the 1983 Act was selective in the manner in which it introduced and enforced patient's rights. Little was done about the admission procedure for example, rather more about consent and MHRTs, and some changes made in the way in which mentally abnormal offenders were dealt with. Even so, and as shown throughout the various chapters, many features of the Act would benefit from further legal consideration. Some may require minor changes, tidying up existing legal anomalies, others require something more extensive – in the area of consent for example the procedure and manner itself could be developed. Others may require something more substantial involving greater deliberation and shifts in the underlying concepts. The opportunities are there, for it is unlikely that we shall have to wait a further 25 years before new legislation is introduced.

The possibilities are endless. Such changes as are thought necessary could still be justified on the principle of equity, for mental patients have rather less than provided for other deviant groups in the way of rights. Appeals procedures prior to compulsory detention are a case in point, so too are the semi-indeterminate sentences for the mentally abnormal offenders. There is still much to do. There may be possibilities for extending the rights of patients above the principle of equity; all patients in all types of hospitals deserve a rather better deal, whether it be in the type of drugs prescribed or whatever.

There are however limitations, some of which have been mentioned above. Notably, that all rights movements, and particularly the type of movement used in mental health, rely as much on the integrity of those enforcing the rules as on those whose rights are violated being able to seek redress. The other serious defect is that this type of movement hardly touches questions relating to patient care, of its quality and extent. It cannot protect patients from government decisions to close mental hospitals, from providing too little money for the psychiatric services, from the occasional poor quality of psychiatric staff, whose training, expertise and commitment to their patients may be less than desirable. It cannot protect patients from overenthusiastic claims that certain types of psychiatric treatments will assist them when the evidence is to the contrary, from cursory treatment by medical and allied staff or from the unreliability of psychiatric diagnosis. Yet somehow one feels it ought, or rather that patient care of that quality ought somehow to be considered.

Of course the Mental Health Act Commission has a responsibility to look at some of these questions, but whether it will pursue them vigorously is an altogether different matter. It was created as a watchdog to monitor the quality of mental health services, able to investigate complaints and inspect mental health facilities. In carrying out its duties, the Commission will not be concerned with the question of whether a patient should have been detained when he wasn't, or should continue to be detained – the latter being the function of the MHRT. Neither will it inspect and report on the general services that are available in psychiatric hospitals, for this is the function of the Advisory Services and the Development Team for the Mentally Handicapped. (Jones, 1984). Most of all, the Commission does not have power to enforce its recommendations, that power being retained by the Secretary of State. One can perhaps see why MIND favoured a patient-advocacy scheme which, in its view, would have greater effect. This of course fits into MIND's general scheme of things, which is founded on the basis of legal theory yet containing all the strength and limitations of that approach.

There is a second possibility, not an alternative but complementary; it involves strengthening the existing bodies, granting them new powers and (dare I say it?) injecting them with new personnel. Many committees such as the Community Health Councils already exist but remain largely impotent acting on the bidding of the medical profession. They rarely initiate, rarely condemn, and rarely provide more than an element of respectability to existing structures. Key committees in mental hospitals do not dilute the power of the medical profession, for the claims of clinical responsibility from medical practitioners seem to be used successfully to thwart attempts to intervene.

Yet these committees have some responsibility for patient care, as well as direct responsibility for certain aspects of the day-to-day running of the hospital. Yet, too often, we provide the structures and go some way to providing the committees but then give too little in the way of power and influence. If changes can be made in social services departments where independent members are drafted to influential committees and panels, so too could there be changes in mental health services. All that is required is the political commitment to do so and the willingness to cope with the ensuing wrath of the medical profession which would see this as a further erosion of its power and influence (which it most surely would be).

The protection of patients' rights, narrowly defined as covering claim rights developed out of legal statutes, is one way of expressing concern for patients. It is not the only one by any means, although it offers a unique provision. It offers the possibility of legal redress, which may involve damages and compensation, and offers too a standard of professional behaviour which ought not be violated. It offers the resources of other professional bodies, although at the same time becomes dependent on the willingness of those additional bodies to consider the case. It does not, or cannot, deal with endless questions related to the day-to-day management of patients, those endless bureaucratic questions and those endless personal contacts which added together make up the quality of patient care. The difference between the good or the bad mental hospital has much to do with the preservation of rights but as much (if not more) to do with the way the hospital is administered and the confidence promoted and the quality of the interaction between patients and staff (as well, of course, with the quality and expertise of the staff). No patients' rights campaign can deal with these, nor any centralised commission. If rights are to be defined more generously, to include the broadest and widest aspects of patient care, greater involvement is required from the existing bodies whose task so defined is to rubberstamp professional decisions.

Section IV

Conclusion

CHAPTER 11

Assessment and conclusion

To repeat an earlier point: the 1983 Act is a piece of reforming legislation rather than a radical one. It seeks to amend, modify and update existing practices whilst retaining the basic philosophy established by the 1959 Act. It should be adjudged on that basis. Yet, in some respects, it is innovative; the consent procedures, for example, break new ground and the Mental Health Act Commission is new (albeit modelled on the Commissioners in Lunacy, established in the nineteenth century and their successors the Board of Control). Mostly it tidies up anomalies and attempts to provide detained patients with more rights without, of course, committing the government to a great deal of additional expenditure. Its major achievement is I think to create a new ethos, a new style and a more up-to-date approach. It also I think provides hope for the future, hope that patients will be recognised as people of some worth whose opinions matter or have to be considered, and hope too that mental health legislation will be updated along similar lines and with greater regularity.

I do not wish simply to add detailed criticisms to the failures of the legislation, for no Act of Parliament remains without criticism and no Act would be expected to include everything. Rather I wish to expand upon two or three topics which require further emphasis. Again, these are not intended to suggest priority but have been selected because they pose some of the most intractable sets of problems. We can begin by taking a general overview of mental disorder, the law and psychiatry.

The first point to make is that mental health or mental disorder is a multimillion pound industry. It provides employment for countless thousands of people in medical and allied professions whether it be the

187

medical practitioners themselves, the nursing staff, administrators, domestics or whatever. Slightly less direct employment for others including those in the drug companies, hospital supplies research and academic research, to name but a few. The structures, social and economic, are sophisticated and immense, the career possibilities often heartening and the content of ideas flowing in and around those structures sometimes interesting and occasionally profound. Yet when one looks at the intellectual foundations upon which those structures are built they appear disturbingly fragile, and the success rates poor.[1]

It is not all doom and gloom of course. There are certain modest achievements in what Clare (1983) refers to as the amelioration and reduction of certain psychotic symptoms for some patients but those achievements are in every sense of the word modest compared to the enormous input. Yet, strangely enough, the most enduring achievement is not something often mentioned in the psychiatric textbooks: that of providing asylum to a number of people who require and need care, consideration and attention to help them through difficult periods of their lives. (It is not often mentioned because the term 'asylum' is no longer fashionable, the medically orientated term 'mental hospital' is preferred.) This seems to be one of the reasons why the structures are maintained: we need a system to provide asylum for some, and perhaps partial asylum for others who can be maintained in the community. Another such reason for maintaining these structures is that mentally disordered persons present themselves as a large and severe social problem lying outside the general ambit of the criminal law, but as sufficient of a social and public nuisance to warrant control. Psychiatry for all sorts of reasons, (some altruistic, some less so) has claimed responsiblity for these patients and is permitted or encouraged to do so. It may be, in Scull's (1982) terms, the emperors of the mental hospital turn out to have no clothes but until the nakedness is perceived the multimillion pound industry will continue. The sadness is however that questions directed towards the intellectual foundations of that industry are rarely asked and, if they are, are seen as subversive in some way.

Be that as it may, the duty of Parliament is to control and direct that industry through the law, whether through mechanisms which allow certain drugs to be marketed or through the more direct forms of control and direction as with the 1983 Act. The law rarely promotes social changes, more often than not it follows shifts in opinions or changes in the sociodemographic structures. Yet, curiously enough, in the case of the 1983 Act it has tended to ignore one such shift, that of the growth and importance of the elderly who are (more than any other group) desperately in need of that form of asylum provided by psychiatrists and the mental hospitals. In turn, the law has retained a view of mental disorder which is becoming outdated, or if not then being left behind by social events. It seems to me that there are assumptions built into the 1983 Act where the aim is to control a certain type of mentally disordered patient – an ideal type, as it were – of young or youngish people suffering from affective disorders such as schizophrenia or the manic depressive conditions and possibly criminal to boot. Whilst there is no doubt these patients remain a problem, they are no longer the major one nor will they be in the future. Like it or not, the elderly will assume greater and greater importance (but then Sir Aubrey Lewis made this point as far back as 1945). 'I think it is pretty clear where all this leads. We must regard the mental disorders of the elderly as likely to be responsible within the next 30 years for the bulk of the patients admitted to mental hospitals' (in Post, 1983). In an epidemiological study of admission rates in London, Norris notes 'In the course of their lives out of every 1,000 males only 8 will be admitted for schizophrenia; 8 for manic depressive including involution psychosis but 21 for the psychosis of old age. The figures for females are rather higher: out of 1,000 there will be 10 for schizophrenia, 14 for affective psychosis and 28 for senile psychosis' (quoted in Post, 1983, p. 280). To say that most observers know this, are aware of this and still do little about it is only part of the problem. To add further that the 1983 Act did little to help provide relief for the elderly is another area needing to be considered.

There is the other perennial dispute relating to the extent and amount of money spent on psychiatric provisions for the elderly. These questions lie outside the boundary of that to be considered here which is directed more towards the provisions of the legislation, although I am suggesting a serious defect in the legislation; it could have promoted additional services had Parliament so wished. Unfortunately, the elderly have few supporters outside their main pressure groups such as Age Concern and the like. Organisations such as MIND or professional representatives from the medical and legal profession rarely take up the cudgels on their behalf, with one or two notable exceptions. Modern psychiatry has tended to neglect the elderly preferring to concentrate on the acute patients. In fact psychiatry, like so many other medical specialisms tends to avoid the chronic patients altogether, whether they be the elderly or the younger mentally impaired. Chronicity appears not to fit the magic derived from high technology modern medicine where diagnosis, treatment and a constant turnover of patients is more the order of the day. The demented elderly with a chronic condition and a poor prognosis, dominated by questions of care and management do not fit into the magic fashioned by the technological world. We are back to the multimillion pound industry argument again where I am suggesting that care and management should be its major justification, and if so the elderly certainly qualify for that.

Yet, irrespective of the preferences of psychiatrists, the discipline will inevitably become more and more dominated by concerns of the elderly. The sociodemographic changes are too important to avoid it. In spite of Sir Aubrey Lewis' warnings, there seems a reluctance to admit that these demands are imminent. In 1981 there were still only about 120 consultant psychiatrists in Britain with a special interest in the elderly, mainly in Scotland and the South East of England and, of those, only 41% could be considered to be working full-time as psychogeriatricians (the remainder as half time or working only occasionally). This situation may be bad in Britain but is apparently worse elsewhere (see Post, 1983, p. 291).

How then should the law respond, aside that is from the provision of extra services. In the spirit of the type of legislation contained within the 1983 Act, I suggest the following: most elderly patients are informal and not therefore covered by the consent procedures (nor, for the same reason, are they covered by the tribunal procedure). Yet some, with certain levels of assistance, could be helped to live in the community. (Ovenstone & Bean, 1981). Guardianship procedures are often too cumbersome and formal whilst the Court of Protection deals only with patients' financial affairs, not with questions of care and management. One possibility is to insist that all long-stay elderly patients, particularly informal ones come before a MHRT after a given time, say 18 months or so to have their cases reassessed. This would encourage at least the hospital authorities to produce programmes of care and management. Another is to enlarge the provisions whereby surrogates are appointed so that all long-stay elderly patients have someone available to protect their interests, perhaps a lawyer or someone of similar standing.

Another priority is to re-examine Section 47 of the 1948 National Assistance Act. It seems to be used relatively infrequently, about 200 times in England and Wales each year but there are no central records kept and that figure may be inaccurate. Its use was thought to be declining up to 1979 but the Chronically Sick and Disabled Persons Act 1970 imposed a duty on local authorities to seek out people qualifying for help and this, together with the Housing and Homeless Persons Act 1977, might have pushed the numbers up since then (Greengross, 1982). The problem is that Section 47 can be used to bypass the normal mental health procedure.

It will be remembered that Section 47 says patients may be forcibly placed in institutional care to secure the necessary care and attention if they are (*a*) suffering from grave chronic disease, or being aged or physically incapacitated are living in insanitary conditions and (*b*) are unable to devote to themselves, and are not receiving from other persons, care and attention. Under the 1948 Act the local authority may then apply to a magistrates' court for an order committing that person to institutional care, having given 7 days notice to him or someone in charge of him. The maximum period for such an order is 3 months but it can be renewed (however very few elderly people, about 1 in 5, return to their homes after such an order is made, Greengross (1982)). The 1951 National Assistance (Amendment) Act changes the requirements, allowing an emergency order to be made committing the person immediately to care on the authority of the court. This order lasts for 3 weeks, during which time the local authority can apply for the order to be extended to the normal 3 months period. Needless to say, the criteria used are obscure, there are few legal safeguards and there is no possibility of legal aid being granted at the magistrates' court hearing.

It is suspected that Section 47 may be used, and perhaps increasingly as an adjunct to mental health legislation – most of those qualifying for Section 47 are likely to have a form of mental disorder anyway. On balance there may be some value in retaining it, but with one condition: that a closer examination be made of its use before a judgement is made. Section 47, alongside so much else relating to the elderly, needs careful scrutiny and constant evaluation. These changes may go some way to improving the current position of the elderly in the mental health services although without a wholesale re-think of the services generally, they will do little more than scratch the surface. In fact the time is right for a Royal Commission on the services of the elderly, with special reference to the Mental Health services. That Commission would have the advantage of looking at the range of services and help plan for the likely influx of elderly patients shortly to descend upon us.

The second issue I wish to touch upon was examined briefly in Chapter 6 on the mentally abnormal offender. It was suggested there that patients faced two control systems, that of the penal system and that of the mental health services. Some were sent direct to mental hospitals; other patients could, and sometimes should, be transferred from the penal system to the mental health system – but not the other way in the first instance – whenever and wherever necessary. It was also suggested that the penal system as currently constituted was unable to care for the mentally disordered (which, for these purposes, mean the prisons) yet transfer was necessary if patients were to receive appropriate treatment. In that chapter I suggested that opposition to such transfers and the use of hospital orders came from the psychiatric services whereby the right was claimed to treat those patients of its own choosing. That is mental hospital staff objected to patients being foisted upon them by the courts or by the prison service, many of whom would be regarded as untreatable or, if not, then sufficiently disruptive to upset the hospital routine. In spite of the advantages to the patient in terms of receiving appropriate treatment, it was also suggested that such patients as there were might oppose the making of an order or a transfer. They would tend to see it as being caught in a trap. Once in the mental health system, they are faced with the indeterminate sentence, their discharge being dependent on their progress in treatment and not according to a sentence fixed at the outset by the court. That they may and often do spend longer under mental health regimes than in the prison is to them a matter of some importance.

An opportunity to examine the question was given to the Butler Committee who, regrettably, passed it by. They were not concerned, they said, with challenging basic philosophies but with recommending changes according to existing ones, and presumably saw this as a challenge to the basics. Yet one can see how and why the patient may be reluctant to accept a hospital order or transfer or indeed be reluctant to promote such orders. Assume he was serving a 6 month sentence or would have served such a sentence had he been sent to prison (with his earliest date of release 4 months hence). Unless he lost remission, or commited further offences whilst in prison he could expect to be released on that date. Once inside the mental health system, he can be prevented from being released by the renewal of this hospital order or transfer direction. Of course, there are provisions for appeals under the MHRTs and it is also true that hospitals will not wish to keep patients longer than necessary. It is equally true that the patient is receiving psychiatric treatment appropriate to his condition which he would not have received otherwise. We can accept all this yet still regard a system as unfair when, as a result of a prison sentence (possibly of short duration), the patient is detained in a hospital for a great deal longer. There are also the other questions about the effectiveness of the treatments (that is, would the patient have improved if left to himself anyway), the dangerousness of such treatments including their long-term effects, and the so-called labelling effect resulting from a compulsory admission.

One suggested solution is for the courts to sentence on the basis of proportionality or retribution where the offender serves a sentence according to deserts. This may be all very well for offenders going direct to a hospital but does not meet the point for those transferred to a hospital. Even then, sentences based on proportionality would not prevent the offender being detained at the end of his sentence under civil commitment procedure if the hospital managers considered further detention to be necessary. Once inside the mental health system the offender comes within its dictates. Yet the advantage of proportionality is to force a decision at the end of the patient's sentence as to the appropriateness of extending his detention in hospital and allowing the patient to appear before a MHRT when legally permitted. That may be to his advantage but I confess to seeing no solution to that where patients are transferred.

However, to complicate matters further, patients on a hospital order occasionally find themselves at an advantage over their contempories receiving a prison sentence. While they risk the possibility of extended periods in the hospital, the truth of the matter is that many abscond and little is done about it. The open-door policy of modern mental hospitals makes them ill-suited to receive such patients, or rather hospitals interpret their duties in ways which emphasise the voluntary nature of treatment. Hospitals dislike formal controls, unless imposed by themselves of course, and dislike being answerable to outside authorities. The result is a less-than-satisfactory outcome, whether for the courts who believe the offender is being provided with treatment under reasonably secure conditions, or for the probation services where offenders are detained in hospital as a condition of their probation or for the offender and hospital authorities alike. Conditions are quite different of course for offenders in Special Hospitals or Regional Secure Units where the converse applies, for they are likely to face additional detention. Here we are talking of those on hospital orders going to ordinary mental hospitals.

The Butler Committee considered the problem but passed this one over as well. It said that when a patient who is subject to a hospital order absconds it should be for the responsible medical officer to seek to have him returned to the hospital. The Committee thought that this proposal comes closest to meeting the practical needs of the present-day hospital without giving rise to serious risk to the public. It thought 'the doctor was best able to judge the prospective risk if the patient remains at large and to what extent the patient might be willing or able to respond to medical treatment should he be returned' (HMSO, 1975). I wish this were so; even if it were it comes dangerously close to making a mockery of the whole procedure. That is, an offender is sent to a hospital to receive treatment (having committed an imprisonable offence), absconds and nothing is done about it on the grounds that he is neither a risk to the public nor will respond to treatment. (It is often suggested that there are parallels with a probation order, for the court has no control over the manner in which the probation officer runs his caseload. The difference is the Court has imposed a custodial sentence when making a hospital order even though, for convenience, it is called something else.) The Butler Committee's proposal on this, as with many others, was a further attempt to avoid upsetting those in the mental hospitals and seeking always to leave them with the ultimate choice and decision.

Again I confess to seeing no simple answer where one control system detains on the basis of deserts, which by their very nature involve sentences fixed by the Court, and the other on the basis of a disease which is by its nature less predictable and its natural history dependent on factors which are often unknown. I think a start could be made to make hospital authorities more accountable and, if the suggestion in Chapter 6 is accepted, more amenable to the court's wishes. This will not necessarily provide a solution but it will show where future developments are likely.

The third and final topic concerns the legislation itself. Its history has yet to be written, as opposed to the formal sequences of events provided by the government, and other official publication flowing from those events. That history may unearth some new and interesting facts about the influence of pressure groups, the influence of more shadowy figures such as civil servants who appear less prominent yet who may have exerted great influence. It may also show the influence of various government advisors who not only helped select the Chairman of the initial Mental Health Act Commission but its members too. It may show too the extent to which government and various professional bodies interacted to produce the final version. Then there is the extent of parliamentary time, to consider and the composition of the parliamentary committees. The 1983 Act provides an opportunity for a study within the framework of the sociology of law, for this piece of legislation offers a unique chance to enlarge our understanding of such matters. A study of the official Parliamentary Debate shows how the legislation provides a fascinating mixture of political manoeuvering mixed with the public face of moral hectoring together with a genuine concern for the position of a vulnerable group, the mental patients. It shows too how party antagonisms can occasionally be put aside producing what the French would call 'alliances against nature', and also how some Parliamentary Members, whose views on political matters may be extreme, show rare sympathies when pulled out of the party battleground to make less predictable judgments. Conversely others, whose public sympathies have been frequently displayed, appeared less sympathetic on this issue.

Then there remains the question of whether the legislation will work. This is largely an empirical question, the results to be determined by empirical inquiry. Consent procedures for example need to be examined, so too do the activities of the Mental Health Act Commission, and the tribunals to name but a few. These inquiries would provide evidence for assessments about the effectiveness of these parts of the Act. There are many other areas which could profitably be examined. No doubt we shall all be flooded with codes of practice from the Commission but the implementation of these codes will be of more importance. Yet, for the Act to be effective, it requires more than empirical inquiries and codes of practice: it requires a considerable amount of goodwill. That can only come from the medical and allied professions whose daily task it is to be in contact with the patients and to implement many of the procedures. If they are hostile to the general principles of the Act, it could quickly be sabotaged. There are signs that some hostility exists where psychiatric staff resent attempts to scrutinise their activities, and the social work fiasco (so described by a Committee of MPs) relating to social work training bodes ill for the future.

Goodwill is required too from the lawyers. It was said earlier that most lawyers had until the early 1980s showed little interest in mental health matters. Suddenly mental health has become legally fashionable. Fashions tend, however, to be unstable. Might it not be that lawyers, finding few commercial rewards in mental health, depart for more lucrative pastures leaving a few stalwarts to bear the brunt of it all? If so it will be very sad indeed yet there seems a distinct possibility that it will happen.

It is likely that the 1983 Act will be amended frequently to be followed by more substantial legislation at a later date. Perhaps new legislation will change the direction again, pointing to different ways of looking at things. As they stand at present we seem to be witnessing the decline of the mental hospital and the growth of various forms of community care. That too may change to produce something different again. That is for the future; in the meantime we must work with what we have which, for all its defects, is the product of a great deal of contemporary thinking.

NOTES

Chapter 1

1 In January 1975 the then Labour Government announced its intention to review the 1959 Mental Health Act. An Interdepartmental Committee was set up to undertake the review and reported in 1976. That consultative document '*A review of the Mental Health Act 1959*' (HMSO, 1976) invited comments on its proposals. The public response was contained in a White Paper '*Review of the Mental Health Act 1959*' (Cmnd. 7320). With the change in Government, the Conservatives published their own White Paper '*Reform of Mental Health Legislation*' (Cmnd. 8405) and introduced a Bill which subsequently became the Mental Health (Amendment) Act 1982. This Act was followed by the consolidating Mental Health Act 1983 which received the Royal Assent on 9 May 1983. Regulations relating to this Act followed. See also Bean, P.T. (1979). The Mental Health Act 1959: rethinking an old problem. *British Journal of Law and Society*, **6**, No. 1, 99–108, for a commentary on the proposal up to the change in government.

2 Official statistics on national data tend not to be good. To supplement these, the three tables below provide data from a census of a mental hospital in Nottingham (Mapperley) taken in 1982. This hospital may not be representative of other hospitals in England and Wales, indeed in many respects it is unusual but has the advantage of operating a comprehensive psychiatric register from which these data are extracted. Table 1 shows the number of admissions and demonstrates the downward trend. Mapperley Hospital serves a large conurbation with a population of roughly half a million people. (I am grateful to the managers of Mapperley Hospital Nottingham for granting permission to use these data, and especially to Professor John Cooper, Professor of Psychiatry, University of Nottingham.)

Table 1. Number of admissions between 1976 and 1981

Year	Number of admissions
1976	1976
1977	1892
1978	1893
1979	1843
1980	1863
1981	1746

For the years 1980 and 1981 there were 130 (or about 7%) and 115 (or 6.6%) admitted patients detained under the Mental Health Act – the 1959 Act as it was then.

196

Table 2 shows the length of stay of the total hospital population of 609 patients at the time of the census.

Table 2. Length of stay of patients

Length of Stay	No. of patients	Percentage
Less than 1 month	88	14.5
Over 1 month, less than 2 months	68	11.2
Over 2 months less than 12 months	110	18.1
Over 1 year less than 5 years	172	28.2
Over 5 years less than 15 years	94	15.4
Over 15 years less than 25 years	32	5.2
Over 25 years	45	7.4
Total	609	100.0

Table 3 shows the diagnosis of patients admitted for the first time over a 5 year period.

Table 3. Diagnosis of first admissions over a 5 year period

Diagnosis	Percentage (rounded up)
Organic psychosis	24
Schizophrenic/paranoid psychosis	11
Affective psychosis	28
Drugs/alcohol	9
Neurosis	28
Other	1
Total	101%

In spite of fears (or claims) that long-stay patients have been turned out of the hospitals in large numbers under the guise of community care, Table 1 shows a large percentage of patients had been in that hospital for over 5 years. Indeed 12.6% had been in for over 15 years although 25.7% had been in for less than 12 months. Table 3 shows a fairly even distribution between organic, affective psychosis and the neuroses. The numbers admitted for drugs/alcohol are high, reflecting an interest in and special facilities for these types of patients in that hospital.

3 It is interesting in this context to note that the influential *Psychiatric Dictionary* (1981, 5th edn, ed. R.S. Campbell, Oxford University Press) does not define mental illness, nor includes it in the Dictionary.

Chapter 3

1 The Section relating to admission for treatment (Section 3) adds an additional twist to the general problem. Section 3 says the grounds for detention are if the patient is suffering from mental illness, severe mental impairment, psychopathic disorder or mental impairment and his mental disorder is of a nature or degree which makes it appropriate for him to receive medical treatment in a hospital. As Hoggett (1984, p. 59) puts it with her usual clarity, 'there is no mention of the mental disorder being appropriate to compel the patient to go'. That is, the law makers must have assumed that whenever the patient was suffering from one of those types of mental disorder sufficient to require hospital treatment it was sufficient also to require compulsory hospital treatment. Surely an unwarranted assumption, but one that remains unchallenged in the current legislation.

Chapter 5

1 Subject to certain conditions, Section 47 of the National Assistance Act 1948 allows the compulsory removal to hospital or elswhere of 'persons who are (a) suffering from grave chronic disease or being aged, infirm or physically incapacitated are living in insanitary conditions and (b) are unable to devote to themselves and are not receiving from other persons proper care and attention'.

Chapter 9

1 Salmond on Torts at p. 227 states 'Breach of statutory duty is a tort in itself . . . If a statute imposes a duty for the protection of particular citizens or a particular class of citizen, it *prima facia* creates at the same time a correlative right vested in those citizens, and *prima facia* therefore they will have the ordinary civil remedy for the enforcement of that right namely on action for damages in respect of any loss occasioned by the violation of it'.

   The other leading law textbook on torts (Clerk & Lindsell) states on p. 59 '. . . the breach of a statute may give use to an action commonly spoken of as an action for breach of statutory duty, which is for most practical purposes the creation of a tort, or a group of torts . . .'.

2 Article 6(1) of the European Convention states

   In the determination of his civil rights and obligations or of any criminal charge against him, everyone is entitled to a fair and public hearing within a reasonable time by an independent and impartial tribunal established by law. Judgment shall be pronounced publicly but the press and public may be excluded from all or part of the trial in the interests of morals, public order or national security in a democratic society, where the interests of juveniles or the protection of the private life of the parties so require, or to the extent strictly necessary in the opinion of the Court in special circumstances where publicity would prejudice the interests of justice. See also Hoggett (1984).

3 Many of these points were introduced by Professor R. Davies to MIND in a seminar given in March 1985.

Reference

Hoggett, B. (1984). *Mental Health Law*, 2nd edn. London: Street & Maxwell.

Chapter 10

1 It is doubtful if any other modern industry operates on such flimsy and uncertainty. Consider the disease classifications: they still remain obscure, so much so that one eminent American psychiatrist Karl Menninger produces and publicly advocates a counsel of despair when he says that classifying psychiatric patients is unscientific and unnecessary since all forms of illness are the same and differ only in degree (Menninger, *et al.* 1963). From distinguished British psychiatrists we are offered something less grandiose and for that reason more incisive. Kendall (1976) for example, reminds us that the study of depression has produced no agreement about the nature of endogenous or reactive depression, whether they are the same or extremes of a continuum. For schizophrenia: is it a number of illnesses and if so how many? Is it one condition with numerous features? No one appears to know.

   Consider diagnosis and treatment: it is not necessary to emphasise the well-known point that inter-rater reliability in diagnosis is no better that would be obtained by chance. On the question of treatment Clare (1983) says that, despite the fact that a substantial number of drug studies have confirmed the powerful effects of the neuroleptic drugs in ameliorating and in many cases eliminating psychotic symptoms in schizophrenia, there is remarkably little evidence to suggest that the cure rate for the disorder has changed very much in the 90 years since Emil Kraeplin first described the condition. Clare has little to be enthusiastic about when considering the effects of the psychotherapies, for he says such therapies are complex, time-consuming and expensive and exercise modest effects in conditions which are relatively benign to begin with.

References

Clare, A. (1983) Treatment and cure in mental illness. In *Mental Illness. Changes and Trends*, ed. P.T. Bean, pp.137–61. John Wiley & Sons.
Kendell, R.E. (1976). *The Classification of Depressive Illnesses*. Oxford: Oxford University Press.
Menninger, K. (1963). *The Vital Balance*. Viking Press.

Chapter 1

Bean, P.T. (1980). *Compulsory Admissions to Mental Hospitals*. Chichester & New York: John Wiley & Sons.

Bean, P.T. (1985). Social control and social theory in secure accommodation. In *Secure Provision*, ed. L. Gostin. London: Tavistock.

Bluglass, R. (1985). The recent Mental Health Act in the United Kingdom: issues and perspectives. In *Psychiatry, Human Rights and the Law*, ed. M. Roth & R. Bluglass. Cambridge University Press.

Curran, W. & Harding, T. (1978). *The Law and Mental Health: Harmonizing Objectives*. Geneva: WHO.

DHSS (1976). *A Review of the Mental Health Act 1959*. London: HMSO,

DHSS (1978). *Review of the Mental Health Act 1959*. London: HMSO, Cmnd 7320.

DHSS (1981). *Reform of Mental Health Legislation*. London: HMSO, Cmnd 8405.

Gostin, L. (1983). *A Practical Guide to Mental Health Law*. London: MIND.

Gostin, L. (1984). *A Review of Secure Accomodation For Mental Patients*. Mimeo.

HMSO (1957). Royal Commission on the law relating to mental illness and mental deficiency 1954–7 (The Percy Commission), Cmnd 169.

HMSO (1975). Report of the Committee on mentally abnormal offenders (The Butler Report). Cmnd 6244.

Hoggett, B. (1984). *Mental Health Law*, 2nd ed. London: Sweet & Maxwell.

Jones, R.M. (1984), *The Mental Health Act 1983*. London: Sweet & Maxwell.

Ovenstone, I. & Bean, P.T. (1981). A medical social assessment of old people's homes in Nottingham. *British Journal of Psychiatry*, **139**, 226–9.

Roth, M. (1985). The historical background: the past 25 years since the Mental Health Act of 1959, (eds), In *Psychiatry, Human Rights and the Law*, ed. M. Roth & R. Bluglass. Cambridge University Press.

Scull, A. (1983), The asylum as community or the community as asylum, In: *Mental Illness: Changes and Trends*, ed. P.T. Bean. Chichester & New York: John Wiley & Sons.

Szasz, T. (1970) *Ideology and Insanity*. London: Pelican.

WHO (1980). *International Classification of Impairment Disabilities and Handicaps*. Geneva: WHO.

Chapter 2

Bean, P.T. (1980). *Compulsory Admissions to Mental Hospitals*. Chichester & New York: John Wiley & Sons.

Bean, P.T. (1986). Social work and mental illness. In Bean P.T. and Whynes D. (eds) *Barbara Wootton: Social Science and Public Policy: Essays in her Honour*. London: Tavistock.

British Association of Social Workers (1976). Review of the 1959 Mental Health Act. *Social Work Today*, **6**, No. 24 (March) pp. 770–1.

DHSS (1983a) *Mental Health Act 1983*.

DHSS (1983b) *Mental Health Act 1983 Approved Social Workers*.LAC (83)7 June.

HMSO (1957). Minutes of evidence to the Royal Commission on the Law Relating to Mental Illness and Mental Deficiency (Day 4). The Percy Commission.

HMSO (1960). Local Authority and Allied Personal Social Services (Seebohm Report) Cmnd 3703.

HMSO (1985). Sixth Report from the Social Service Committee. HC 339. Public Expenditure on the Social Services.

Hoggett, B. (1984). *Mental Health Law*, 2nd edn. London: Sweet & Maxwell.

Jones, R.M. (1984). *The Mental Health Act 1983*. London: Sweet & Maxwell.

Olsen, R. (1983). A critical evaluation of the proposals for training approved social workers. In *Approved Social Work: Principles and Practice*. London, MIND.

Sarteschi. P., Lassaro, G.B., Mauri, M. & Petracca, A. (1985). Mental and social consequences of the Italian Psychiatric Care Act 1978. In *Psychiatry, Human Rights and the Law*, ed. M. Roth & R. Bluglass. Cambridge University Press.

Bean, P.T. (1980). *Compulsory Admissions to Mental Hospitals*. Chichester & New York: John Wiley & Sons.

Bean, P.T. (1985). Social control and social theory in secure accommodation. In *Secure Provision*, ed. L. Gostin. London: Tavistock.

Chapter 3

COHSE (1978). *The Management of Mental Patients*. Mimeo.
Curran, W. & Harding, T. (1978). *The Law and Mental Health: Harmonising Objectives*. Geneva: WHO.
Gostin, L. (1983). *A Practical Guide to Mental Health Law*. London: MIND.
Gostin, L. (1985). *A Review of Secure Provision for Mental Patients*. Mimeo.
HMSO (1926). Royal Commission on lunacy and mental disorder (The Macmillan Commission), Cmnd 2700.
HMSO (1957). Royal Commission on the law relating to mental illness and mental deficiency (The Percy Commission), Cmnd 169.
Hoggett, B. (1984). *Mental Health Law*, 2nd ed. London: Sweet & Maxwell.
Scheff, T. (1964). *Being Mentally Ill*. Chicago: Aldine.
Scull, A. (1979). *Museums of Madness*. London: Allen Lane.

Chapter 4

Bean, P.T. (1980). *Compulsory admissions to Mental Hospitals*. Chichester & New York: John Wiley & Sons.
Berry, G. & Orwin, A. (1966). No fixed abode. *British Journal of Psychiatry*, **112**, 1019–25.
HMSO (1957). Royal Commission on the law relating to mental illness and mental deficiency 1954–7 (The Percy Commission), Cmnd 169.
HMSO (1975). Report of the Committee on mentally abnormal offenders (The Butler Report), Cmnd 6244.
Hoggett, B. (1984). *Mental Health Law*, 2nd ed. London: Sweet & Maxwell.
Kelleher, M.J. & Copeland, J.R. (1972). Compulsory psychiatric admissions by the police. *Medicine, Science and the Law*, **12**, (3) 220–4.
Mountney, G. Fryers, T. & Freeman, H.L. (1969). Psychiatric emergencies in an urban borough. *British Medical Journal*, **1**, 478–500.
Parliamentary Debates on the Mental Health Act, 18 October 1982.
Rassaby, E. & Rogers, A. (1986). *Psychiatric Referrals from the Police*. London: MIND.
Sims, A. & Symonds, R.L. (1975). Psychiatric referrals from the police. *British Journal of Psychiatry*, **127**, 171–8.
Walker N. & McCabe S. (1973). *Crime and Insanity in England*. Vols 1 & 2. Edinburgh University Press.

Chapter 5

Bean, P.T. (1980). *Compulsory Admissions to Mental Hospitals*. Chichester & New York: John Wiley & Sons.
DHSS (1978). Review of the Mental Health Act 1959, Cmnd 7320.
DHSS (1983). Mental Health Act 1983 Memorandum on Part 1 VI, VIII and X.
Gostin, L. (1983). The ideology of entitlement. In *Mental Illness: Changes and Trends*, ed. P.T. Bean. Chichester & New York: John Wiley & Sons.
HMSO (1957). Royal Commission on the law relating to mental illness and mental deficiency 1954–7 (The Percy Commission), Cmnd 169.
HMSO (1975). Report of the Committee on mentally abnormal offenders (The Butler Report), Cmnd 6244.
HMSO (1983). The mental health (Hospital Guardianship and Consent to Treatment) Regulations No.893 (H93/1179).
Hoggett, B. (1984). *Mental Health Law*, 2nd ed. London: Sweet & Maxwell. *Social Work Today* (1985). Concern mounts over the use of guardianship. 15 July 1985.

Chapter 6

Ashworth, A. & Gostin, L. (1985). Mentally disordered offenders and the sentencing process. In *Secure Provision*, ed. L. Gostin, pp. 211–35. London: Tavistock.

Bean, P.T. (1981). *Punishment: a Philosophical and Criminological Enquiry*. Oxford: Martin Robertson.

Bowden, P. (1985). Psychiatry and dangerousness: a counter renaissance? In *Secure Provision*, ed. L. Gostin, pp. 265–87. London: Tavistock.

COHSE (1977). *The Management of Violent or Potentially Violent Patients*. Confederation of Health Service Employees.

Dell, S. (1980). The transfer of Special Hospital Patients to the NHS hospitals. *Special Hospital Research Unit Report*, No. 16.

DHSS (1975). *Better Services for the mentally ill*. Cmnd 6233, London: HMSO.

DHSS (1976). *The Management of Potentially Violent Patients*. HC 76(11).

DHSS (1980). *Report of the review of Rampton Hospital*. Cmnd 8073.

Foucult, M. (1978). About the concept of the 'dangerous individual' in 19th century legal psychiatry. *International Journal of Law Psychiatry*, 1 (1) 1–18.

Gostin, L. (1985). *A Review of Secure Provision for Mental Patients*. Mimeo.

Hamilton, J.R. (1985). The Special Hospitals. In *Secure Provision*, ed. L. Gostin, pp. 84–125. London: Tavistock.

HMSO (1974). Report of the working party on security in NHS hospitals.

HMSO (1975). Report of the Committee on mentally abnormal offenders (The Butler Report). Cmnd 6244.

HMSO (1982). Parliamentary Debates. Special Standing Committee on the Mental Health (Amendment) Bill, Lords.

HMSO (1985). Sixth Report of the Social Services Committee. House of Commons, paper 339.

Hoggett, B. (1984). *Mental Health Law*, 2nd ed. London: Sweet & Maxwell.

Jones, R.M. (1984). *The Mental Health Act 1983*. London: Sweet & Maxwell.

Wootton, B. (1959). *Social Science and Social Pathology*. London: George Allen & Unwin.

Chapter 7

Bean, P.T. (1980). *Compulsory admissions to Mental Hospitals*. Chichester & New York: John Wiley & Sons.

Clare, A. (1983). Treatment and Cure in Mental Illness. In *Mental Illness Changes and Trends*, ed. P.T. Bean, pp. 137–62. Chichester & New York: John Wiley & Sons.

DHSS (1983). Circular HN (83)37.

Faulder, C. (1985). *Whose Body Is It?* London: Virago Press.

Fennel, P. (1977). The Mental Health Review Tribunal; a question of imbalance. *British Journal of Law and Society*, No.2, 186–219.

Gostin, L. (1983). *A Practical Guide to Mental Health Law*. London: MIND.

Gostin, L., Rassaby, E. & Buchan, A. (1984). *Mental Health: Tribunal Procedure*. London: Oyez Longman.

HMSO (1957) Royal Commission on the law relating to mental disorder and mental deficiency (The Percy Report) Cmnd 169.

HMSO (1975). Report of the Committee on mentally abnormal offenders. (The Butler Report), Cmnd 6244.

Hoggett, B. (1984). *Mental Health Law*. 2nd ed. London: Sweet & Maxwell.

Peay, J. (1982). Mental Health Review Tribunals and the Mental Health (Amendment) Act. *Criminal Law Review*, pp. 779–94.

Scull, A. (1983). The asylum as community or the community asylum in *Mental Illness: Changes and Trends*, ed. P.T. Bean, pp. 329–50. New York: John Wiley & Sons.

Chapter 8

Bean, P.T. (1980). *Punishment: a Philosophical and Criminological Enquiry*. Oxford: Martin Robertson.

Bean, P.T. (1985). Social control and social theory in secure accommodation. In *Secure Provision*, ed. L.O. Gostin pp. 288–306. London: Tavistock.

Bradley, F.H. (1927). *Ethical Studies*. Oxford: Clarendon Press.

Bridges P.K. (1984). Psychosurgery and the Mental Health Act Commission. *Bulletin of the Royal College of Psychiatrists*, August 1984, pp. 146–8.

DIISS (1978). *Review of the Mental Health Act 1959*. Cmnd 7320,

DHSS (1983). *Mental Health (Hospital Guardianship and Consent to Treatment)*. Regulations SI 893, also DHSS (1983) *Phasing in of Consent to Treatment Regulations*. HN(85)35.

Faulder, C. (1985). *Whose Body Is It?* London, Virago press.

Gordon, R. & Verdun-Jones, S. (1983). The right to refuse treatment. *International Journal of Law and Psychiatry*, **6** (1) 57–73.

Gostin, L.O. (1979). The merger of incompetency and certification: the illustration of unauthorised medical contact in psychiatric consent. *International Journal of Law and Psychiatry*, **2**, 127–69.

Gostin, L.O. (1982). Compulsory treatment in psychiatry: some reflections on self determination, patient competency and professional expertises. *Poly Law Review*, **7** (182), 83–93.

Gostin, L.O. (1983). *A Pratical Guide to Mental Health Law*. London: *MIND*.

HMSO (1957). Royal Commission on the law relating to mental illness and mental deficiency 1954–7. (The Percy Commission), Cmnd 169.

HMSO (1975). Report of the Committee on mentally abnormal offenders (The Butler Report), Cmnd 6244.

HMSO (1982) Special standing committee, mental health (amendment) bill. (Lords) 1982 10 May 1982–29 June 1982.

Hoggett, B. (1984). *Mental Health Law*, 2nd edn. London: Sweet & Maxwell.

Kaufman, C.L., Roth, L.H., Lidz, C.W. & Miesel, A. (1981). Informed consent and patient decision making; the reasoning of law and psychiatry. *International Journal of Law and Psychiatry*, **4**, 345–62.

Murphy, J.G. (1979) Therapy and the problem of autonomous consent. *International Journal of Law and Psychiatry*, **2**, 415–30.

National Consumer Council (1983). *Patients' rights*. HMSO.

Spicer, D. (1984). Freeing the child for adoption. In *Adoption: Essays in Social Policy, Law and Sociology*, ed. P.T. Bean, pp. 161–73. London: Tavistock.

Chapter 9

Ashingdane v.U.K. Commission of Human Rights, Application N.8225/78 Report 12 May 1983.

Bean, P.T. (1980). *Compulsory Admissions to Mental Hospitals*. Chichester & New York: John Wiley & Sons.

Bridges, P.K. (1984). Psychosurgery and the mental health act commission. *Bulletin of the Royal College of Psychiatrists*.

British Medical Journal (1889). Editorial, vol. 1, p. London.

HMSO (1976). Royal Commission on civil liability and compensation for personal injury, (The Pearson Commission), Cmnd 7054–1.

Hoggett, B. (1984). *Mental Health Law*, 2nd ed. London: Sweet & Maxwell.

Klein, J. & Glover, S. (1983) Psychiatric malpractice. *International Journal of Law and Psychiatry*, **6** (2) 131–57.

Medical Defence Union (1982). *Annual Report*.

Roth, M. & Bluglass, R. (1985). *Psychiatry, Human Rights and the Law*. Cambridge University Press.

Chapter 10

Adoption Agencies Regulations 1983. No. 1964. London: HMSO.

Bean, P.T. (1980). *Compulsory Admissions to Mental Hospitals*. Chichester & New York: John Wiley & Sons.

Bean, P.T. (1985). Social control and social theory in secure accommodation. In *Secure Accomodation*, ed. L. Gostin, pp. 288–316. London: Tavistock.

Berlin, I. (1969). *Four essays on Liberty*. Oxford: Oxford University Press.

DHSS (1980). Reform of mental health legislation, Cmnd 8405.

Gostin, L. (1979). The merger of incompetency and certification. *International Journal of Law and Psychiatry*, **2** (2), 127–69.

Hoggett, B. (1984). *Mental Health Law*, 2nd edn. London: Sweet & Maxwell.

Lanham, D. (1974). Arresting the insane. *Criminal Law Review*, (Sept.), pp. 518–28.

Jones, R.M. (1984). *The Mental Health Act 1983*. London: Sweet & Maxwell.

Rassaby, A. & Rassaby, E. (1983). An evaluation of the Mental Health Act Commission after one and a half years.

Roth, M. (1985) The historical background: the past 25 years since the Mental Health Act of 1959. In *Psychiatry Human Rights and the Law*, ed. M. Roth & R. Bluglass, pp. 1–7. Cambridge University Press.

Waldron, J. (1984). *Theories of Rights*. Oxford: Oxford University Press.

Chapter 11

Clare, A. (1983). Treatment and cure in mental illness. In *Mental Illness: Changes and Trends*, ed. P.T. Bean, pp. 137–162. Chichester & New York: John Wiley & Sons.

Greengross, S. (1982). Section 47. Age Concern (mimeo).

HMSO (1975). Report of the Committee on mentally abnormal offenders. (The Butler Report), Cmnd 6244.

Kendell, R.E. (1976). *The Classification of Depressive Illness*. Oxford: Oxford University Press.

Ovenstone, I. & Bean, P.T. (1981). A medical social assessment of old peoples homes in Nottingham. *British Journal of Psychiatry*, **139**, 226–9.

Post, F. (1983). Psychogeriatrics as a speciality. In *Mental Illness: Changes and Trends*, ed. P.T. Bean, pp.279–95. John Wiley & Sons.

Index

...ed in the United Kingdom by
...hing Source UK Ltd., Milton Keynes
...3UK00002B/56/P

Printe
Light
13934

Printed in the United Kingdom by
Lightning Source UK Ltd., Milton Keynes
139343UK00002B/56/P